Understanding Fertility Awareness Methods

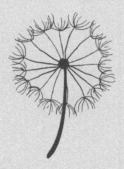

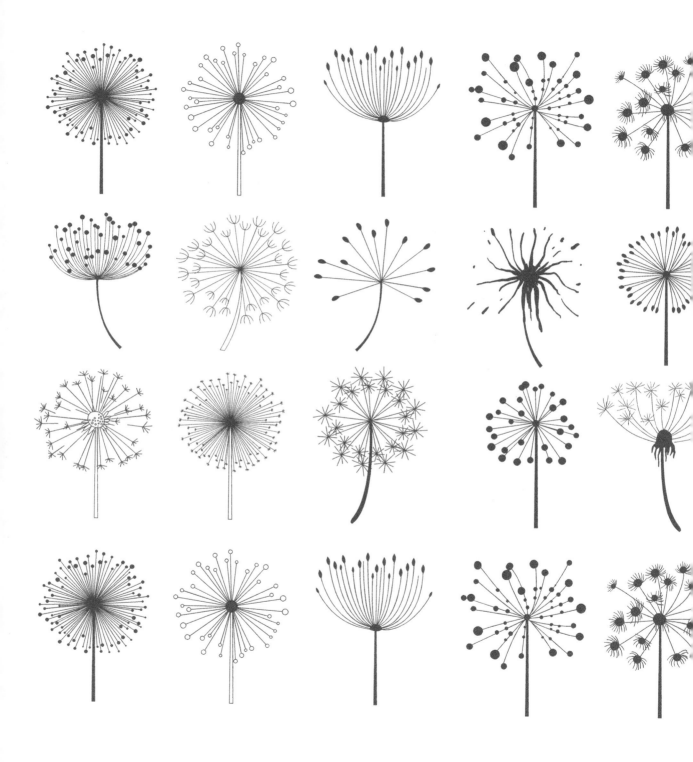

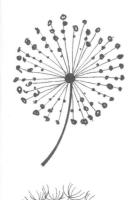

Understanding
Fertility
Awareness
Methods

Gaining Control of
Your Fertility

Rashmi Kudesia, MD, MSc

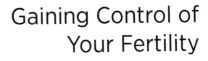

ROCKRIDGE
PRESS

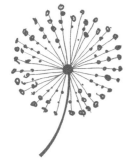

Interior and Cover Designer: Francesca Pacchini
Art Producer: Janice Ackerman
Editor: Mo Mozuch
Production Editor: Andrew Yackira

ISBN: Print 978-1-64739-356-4 | eBook 978-1-64739-357-1
R0

To my daughter, Amara—
I wish so deeply for you to grow up in a world
where every woman, no matter her circumstances,
can access, without question or restriction,
a complete understanding of her body,
feel wonder for the amazing feats it can achieve,
and always have the power of choice over
her reproductive life.

Knowledge is the first step to empowerment.

My words in this book represent just a fraction
of the miraculous beauty of our biology and how families grow,
and I cannot wait to explore it all anew through your eyes . . .

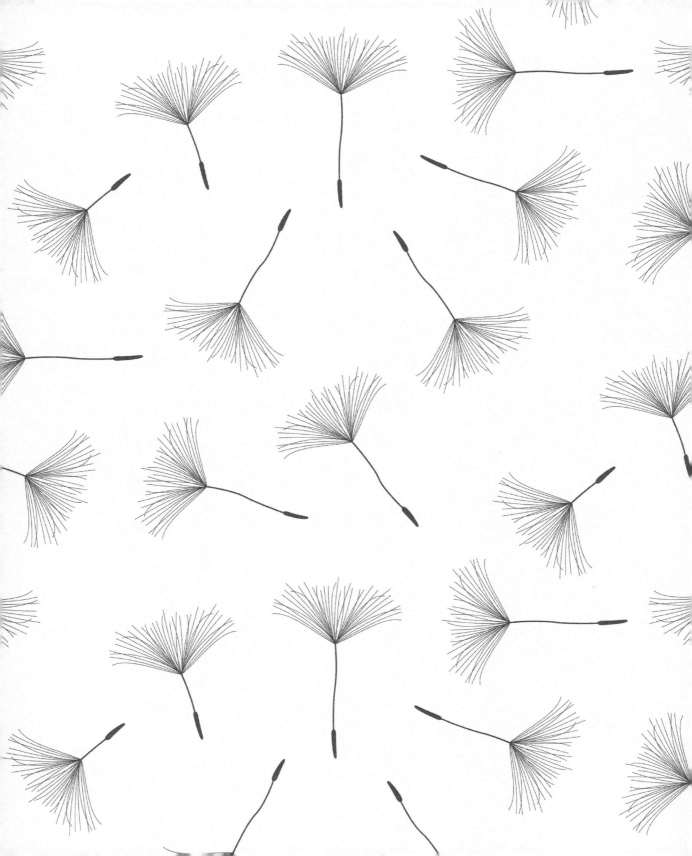

Contents

INTRODUCTION viii

HOW TO USE THIS BOOK xii

Chapter One: Know Your Body, Know Your Cycle 1

Chapter Two: Fertility Complications 13

Chapter Three: Fertility Awareness Methods Explained 35

Chapter Four: Calendar Methods 45

Chapter Five: Tracking Cervical Mucus 53

Chapter Six: Basal Body Temperature 63

Chapter Seven: Charting and Tracking Your FAM 73

Chapter Eight: Tech Support for Your FAM 119

BLANK FAM CHARTS 127

RESOURCES 140

REFERENCES 143

INDEX 147

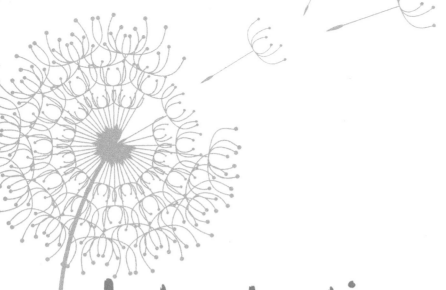

Introduction

My "why" for writing this book is really simple. Day in and day out as a fertility specialist, I take care of women who say things such as, "I wish I had understood all this fertility information years ago," or "I wish I had met you before I had unsuccessful treatment somewhere else." I hear women with treatable diagnoses like polycystic ovary syndrome (PCOS) tell me they were told as teens they would never have children; women with irreversible situations like premature menopause share that their concerns about their changing menstrual cycle were ignored. I hold the hands of women who have had multiple miscarriages and are hoping there is a way to a healthy pregnancy. I have had the privilege of being part of the family-building journey of thousands of women and couples, and though each case is unique, there is one common denominator: women want to know what is going on inside their bodies.

Though there are certainly unknowable realities when it comes to reproductive medicine, with cases of unexplained infertility or recurrent miscarriage, the first step toward pregnancy is figuring out how to conceive. What I hear time and again, though, not just from my patients but from women in so many different contexts in real life or online, from my friends and even my own personal experience, is that we need more access to high-quality scientific advice on how to maximize our fertility. It can feel strangely vulnerable to just have unprotected intercourse and hope that "something happens." And no wonder—without knowing the steps our body should be taking, what we can do to help the conception process along, and when to seek expert input, we are flying blind. So many people do more research on cribs or strollers than on how to actually achieve a healthy pregnancy! Though many women will nonetheless achieve their pregnancy goals without this knowledge, understanding the signs our menstrual cycle sends can assist us in many other health goals in life, and may help us better advocate for and advise our loved ones who might be struggling. Simply put, I advocate strongly for #ReproductiveEmpowerment—every woman having access to medically accurate information that can guide her decision-making about if, when, and how to build a family.

So, out of the many books I hope to write one day, tackling the topic of fertility awareness methods (FAM) has been a passion project for me. I hope it may help some couples not ever need my help in real life—preventing infertility through helping folks achieve pregnancy more efficiently—and I hope it will also help others recognize that they need help and shouldn't delay further. I often tell patients I understand that no one ever really wants to have to come see me. Going to visit a fertility specialist feels very daunting. But just as in real life, my goals in this book are simple: let's review the facts and your options in a thorough way, until you feel comfortable deciding how to move forward. When it comes to FAM, there are so many approaches. We will break it all down in an approachable way, and I hope by the end you will feel empowered and informed along the road of your unique fertility journey.

It saddens me a bit how much of the FAM literature out there paints us physicians as ill-informed or disinterested in women's lived experiences throughout the trying to conceive (TTC) process. It also surprises me how some FAM advocates insist that consistent fertility tracking is just so easy. In my experience, just as women's lives and personalities differ, so, too, does what feels right, comfortable, tolerable, or interesting when it comes to exploring the body's signs and signals. There is no one right way to try or to feel, especially when you have been TTC unsuccessfully for a long time, so I will remind you repeatedly when there are signs that you need help. Seeking that help is not a failure. I regularly see patients who have waited so long that their mental health, or their partner's, or the vitality of their marriage and sex life are struggling. Fertility specialists such as myself train for eleven long years (four years of medical school, four years of residency in obstetrics and gynecology, and three years of fellowship in reproductive endocrinology and infertility) precisely so we can help you with your journey, whether through reassurance, or treatments big or small.

This book can help you understand your reproductive health if you are just hoping to understand your body better, if you are concerned you have a gynecologic issue, if you are worried about your future fertility, if you are hoping to get pregnant soon, or if you have been struggling on the TTC journey. Though pregnancy advice seems to quickly focus on ovulation and timing intercourse, there are many broader facets to our fertility. Your general health impacts your ability to achieve and maintain a healthy pregnancy in numerous ways. It could truly be a separate book, but there are so many lifestyle components that can help improve your outcomes. From the moment you first begin to think about pregnancy, each of these deserves your attention, too:

Diet. Data supports adopting a Mediterranean-style diet, focusing on fresh fruits and vegetables, whole wheat rather than white flour grains, lean poultry or seafood rather than red meat, and overall reduction of processed food.

Beverages. Hydrate! Aim for 60 to 80 ounces of water daily. Avoid the empty sugar in juice and soda, limit caffeine to 200mg daily (typically one cup of coffee), and be mindful of your alcohol intake.

Physical activity. Advice can vary based on your starting fitness level, but try for at least 90 minutes of moderate or high-intensity interval training (HIIT)-style workouts weekly (roughly two to four workouts each week), mixing strength and cardio. I personally love Pilates and barre because they transition seamlessly into early pregnancy with minor modifications.

Medical history. Review any medical diagnoses or medications with your physician. I can't believe how many women come see me actively TTC while on medications contraindicated in pregnancy. Also ensure you are up-to-date on your dental care—unresolved oral disease may worsen fertility and pregnancy outcomes.

Prenatal vitamins. Start this now. Prenatal vitamins help fill in any dietary gaps and are just as much for you as for your baby. Make sure your vitamin has at least 400 micrograms of folic acid, and ideally 200mg of DHA.

Stress management. Whether through exercise, therapy, yoga, acupuncture, meditation, or any other approach, your mental health matters.

In general, I always recommend you speak with your OB/GYN about your pregnancy plans as the time approaches. There are various tests that may be recommended based on your personal or family history, and screening tests you may wish to pursue.

Wherever you are in your fertility journey, I hope that together we get you one step closer to your next goal, and reduce your anxiety along the way. Always remember that you deserve that. As I write this introduction, I am aware of how much more interest society is taking in fertility. I am so happy that more and more folks are talking about reproduction, but the uptick in products and companies trying to capitalize on your questions is also real. So, we'll cut through the noise and help sort out your options. Let's dive in!

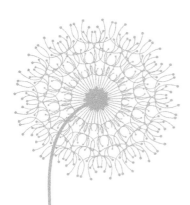

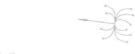

How to Use This Book

This book is meant to help women and couples understand fertility, and how to not only maximize their chances of pregnancy, but also identify when expert evaluation might be indicated. As an educator, I offer the first few chapters to review the intricacies of the reproductive system in a simple way. I hope that understanding the basics of how menstruation, fertility, and pregnancy work will help clarify why certain methods or tests are done, and assist you in interpreting your signs and symptoms throughout your cycle.

We will also talk about the transition off of hormonal contraception and the shift from pregnancy prevention to trying to conceive (TTC). This topic comes up frequently as women try to determine the right timing for stopping birth control, and anticipate not only the return to fertility but their chances of conceiving in any given month. From there, we will dive into the specifics of fertility charting. From simple to more involved methods, from paper charts to smartphone apps, from equipment-free to cutting-edge technology, we will cover it all. The idea is to provide an approachable starting point so you can understand what your options are, and how to get going in tracking your cycles. Though you can use this book at any point in your family-building journey, I hope that many women will find this information when they start thinking about pregnancy, and avoid uncertainty and confusion along the way!

DISCLAIMER

This book discusses how to use fertility awareness methods (FAM) to achieve pregnancy. FAM for pregnancy prevention can be high-risk for failure if not strictly practiced, and we do not offer that level of detail here. Remember, this book is not a substitute for professional medical advice.

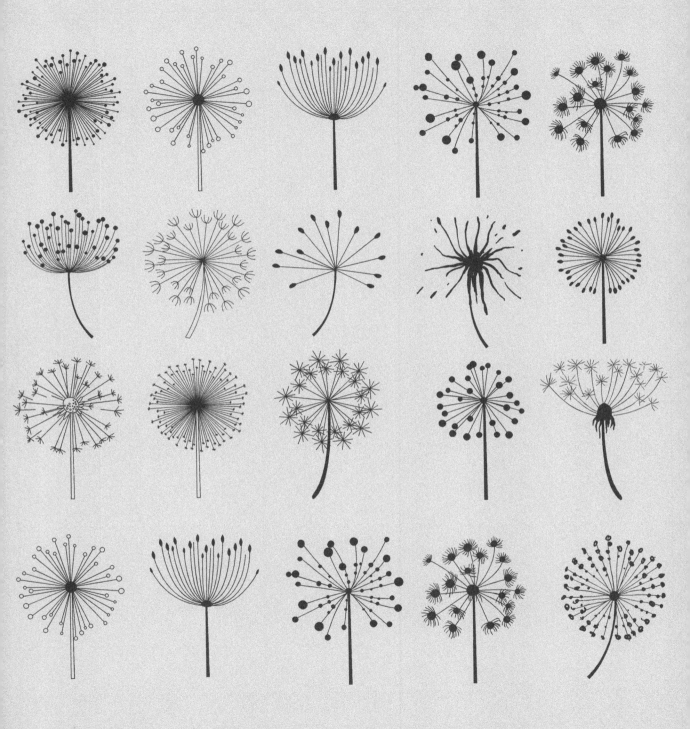

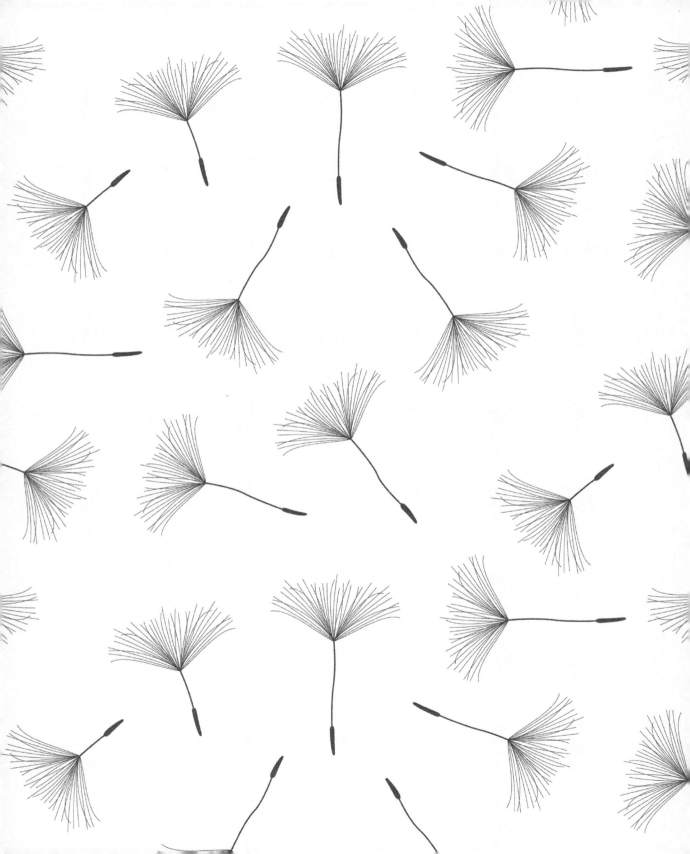

Chapter One

Know Your Body, Know Your Cycle

The first step to fertility awareness is understanding basic repro-
ductive physiology: What are the key components of the menstrual
cycle, and how does each phase relate to fertility and pregnancy?
Though that might sound intimidating, in this chapter, we will
break down the steps of your cycle in simple terms, so that you can
interpret your body's clues to determine if you are ovulating and
when. Listening to what your body is telling you through your menstrual cycle can help you track your reproductive health no matter
where you are in your family-building journey.

In fact, both the American College of Obstetricians and Gynecologists and the American Academy of Pediatrics have endorsed the concept of the menstrual cycle as the "fifth vital sign," alongside your temperature, blood pressure, heart rate, and respiratory rate. This framework highlights the reality that monitoring the regularity, duration, and severity of your period can provide reassurance about your reproductive health or can signal the need for intervention or medical attention.

Since the reproductive system interacts with many other hormones in our bodies, changes in this fifth vital sign can tip us off to a variety of maladies. Knowing your body and your cycle is the key to what I call reproductive empowerment (see #ReproductiveEmpowerment on Instagram), and is the foundation for becoming the best advocate for your reproductive health. Because fertility awareness is a powerful tool for not only optimizing pregnancy but also for monitoring our reproductive health, understanding this basic physiology is critical for every woman and girl, from the first period all the way through menopause.

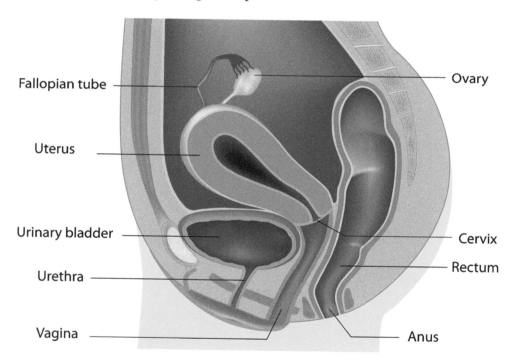

The Menstrual Cycle

Understanding the phases and key events of the menstrual cycle is the foundation of accurately using the fertility awareness method. Though the only evolutionary purpose of the menstrual cycle is to achieve pregnancy, as a species, human beings are relatively inefficient at reproduction: Very few eggs even get a chance at being fertilized, and with each ovulation, the chances of establishing a healthy pregnancy are never more than roughly 25 percent. Unlike men, who produce sperm on an ongoing basis throughout their lives, women are born with all the eggs they will ever have, and the ovaries cannot replace them. The number of available immature eggs peaks at 6 to 7 million halfway through a woman's fetal life and is already down to 1 to 2 million at birth; only 300 to 500 will have the chance to be released in hopes of pregnancy. As fertility specialists, we often discuss the concept of "ovarian reserve," a term that refers to how many eggs remain and their quality.

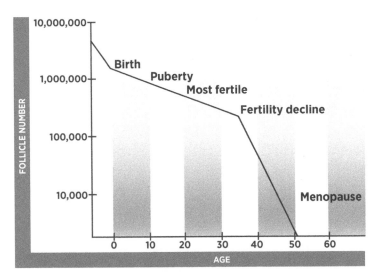

Each menstrual cycle begins with a group of eggs that begin growing, each within its own fluid-filled sac called a follicle. Typically, only one follicle will mature and ovulate, releasing the egg inside. The egg then has a chance of being fertilized, with the resultant embryo implanting into the uterine lining, and progressing into a pregnancy. Due to the hormonal changes accompanying each of these events, our body can demonstrate a pattern of symptoms that signal the procession through these sentinel events. Recognizing these signs is the basis of the fertility awareness method (FAM).

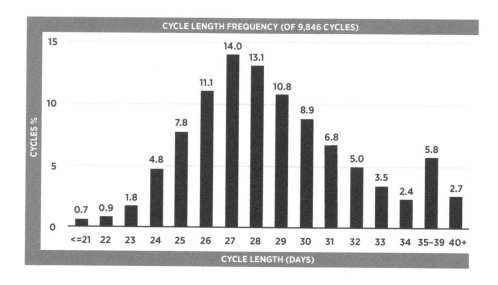

CYCLE LENGTH FREQUENCY (OF 9,846 CYCLES)

The normal menstrual cycle lasts 24 to 38 days, with only a minority of women experiencing the textbook 28-day cycle. The majority of women who experience a regular cycle do ovulate and would almost certainly be undergoing the key steps we will cover here. However, this process of follicular recruitment begins even in women not ovulating regularly, which could range from 15 to 30 percent of the population based on available data. Though we will later discuss the reasons for irregular or absent ovulation, in order to accurately assess one's own ovulatory status, we must first understand the intended sequence of events.

Ovarian Cycle

Reproductive hormones are primarily controlled by an axis of three organs: the hypothalamus and the pituitary gland in the brain, and the ovaries. Each event in the menstrual cycle depends upon the proper secretion and transmission of hormonal messages by these organs.

The hypothalamus's role is primarily to judge the environment to see whether it is an appropriate time to invest the body's important resources into pregnancy. In situations where circumstances seem unfavorable to a healthy pregnancy—due perhaps to an overly restrictive diet or eating disorder, or extreme exercise or stress—the reproductive system shuts down. This system evolved to protect women from getting pregnant during times of famine, unreliable food supply, or war, when pregnancy could be life-threatening. In these situations, no ovulation occurs and the period can stop entirely, which has many long-term negative impacts throughout the body, particularly on bone and heart health.

The ovulatory drive can also be derailed at the level of the pituitary gland, most frequently by benign growths that secrete the hormone prolactin. However, if the hypothalamus and pituitary are functioning normally, the hormones they secrete will guide the ovaries through three phases of activity.

PHASE ONE: FOLLICULAR PHASE

The follicular phase starts with the onset of the period. At this point, the reproductive system should be at baseline, meaning that all follicles are relatively small, usually less than a centimeter. There are waves of follicles starting this process with each cycle, even despite circumstances that typically prevent the cycle from continuing, such as pregnancy, lactation, or hormonal contraception. These follicles produce anti-Müllerian hormone (AMH), the most reliable marker of ovarian reserve. The number of follicles in the monthly cohort decreases with age, and so does the chances of each egg being genetically normal. This means that with increasing age our ovarian reserve continually diminishes.

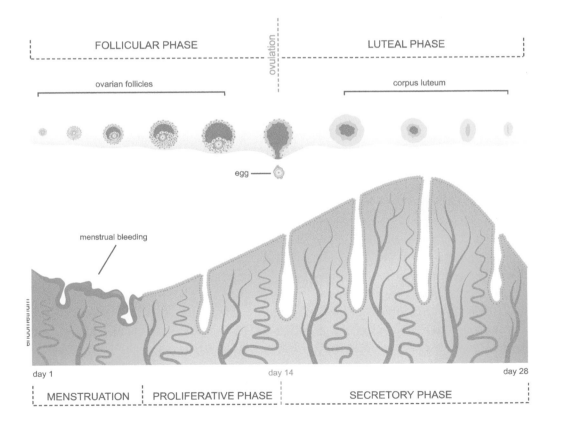

If the hypothalamus perceives a good time for pregnancy, it will emit gonadotropin-releasing hormone (GnRH) in a specific pattern. In response, the pituitary gland will secrete follicle-stimulating hormone (FSH). This stimulates the ovarian follicles with the goal of one follicle becoming dominant and growing larger than the rest. The lower the ovarian reserve, the more FSH must be secreted to induce follicular growth. Some women, especially women in their 40s, will recruit two follicles each month, which is how fraternal twins are spontaneously conceived. The rest of the follicles in the cohort will eventually go through the process of atresia, or dying off.

The follicles secrete estrogen, particularly with growth, and eventually the dominant follicle releases a sustained elevated level of estrogen, triggering ovulation. This process of follicular recruitment and maturation is the most variable part of the cycle, and even among women with a normal menstrual cycle it can range from roughly one to three weeks.

PHASE TWO: OVULATION

Once the dominant follicle has triggered enough estrogen to start the ovulation process, the pituitary gland releases a surge of luteinizing hormone (LH), along with a second, smaller surge of FSH. Within 24 to 36 hours of the LH surge, the egg is released. This day of ovulation, and the five days preceding it, are the only fertile days of the cycle. Later chapters will cover in more detail the symptoms that can help pinpoint the ovulation date, but here is a brief overview.

In the periovulatory (follicular) phase, high estrogen levels can generate symptoms some women experience, such as abdominal bloating, increased libido, and changes to cervical mucus. Others can actually feel pain from the ovulation process, called *mittelschmerz* (German for "middle pain"). A small minority, likely less than 5 percent of women, have light spotting or bleeding at ovulation. Other symptoms women may experience around their ovulation include breast tenderness, nausea, headaches, and fatigue.

PHASE THREE: LUTEAL PHASE

The luteal phase is the time from ovulation to your next period (or from ovulation to a positive pregnancy test!). It is a more reliable window of time at 12 to 14 days, with less variability than the follicular phase. This means that if ovulation definitely occurred, within two weeks you'll either have a period or a pregnancy, a fact that will become critical to properly using FAM.

During the luteal phase, the follicle—now called the corpus luteum—switches from producing estrogen to producing progesterone. Rising progesterone levels after ovulation contribute to the periovulatory symptoms. Since progesterone levels stay high if an embryo implants, they are also responsible for many symptoms experienced in early pregnancy, such as nausea, constipation, and bloating.

Once the egg is ovulated, it is hopefully picked up by the Fallopian tube and will move toward the uterus. If there has been unprotected intercourse and sperm are present in the tube, fertilization may occur with the resulting embryo now moving toward and entering the uterus. If a Fallopian tube has been removed or is blocked, it is possible, though less effective, that the egg can be picked up by the opposite tube. If implantation occurs, it will happen roughly five days after ovulation.

Midway through the luteal phase, the progesterone level peaks. If no implantation has occurred, the corpus luteum will start to lose steam, and the progesterone levels will drop over the next week, triggering the uterine lining to shed in a period. The drop in estrogen and progesterone at this time is responsible for premenstrual symptoms, commonly including mood swings, breast tenderness (yes, again!), food cravings, fatigue, bloating, hormonal migraines, and more. When significant enough, such symptoms can qualify as premenstrual syndrome (PMS) or premenstrual dysphoric disorder (PMDD), which are both valid medical diagnoses that can be treated.

On the other hand, if a pregnancy is beginning, eventually the embryo will secrete the pregnancy hormone beta-human chorionic gonadotropin (β-hCG). The β-hCG supports the corpus luteum so that it can continue making progesterone for roughly six more weeks, until the placenta is established and takes control over hormone production.

LUTEAL PHASE DEFECT: A REAL ENTITY?

Since the late 1940s, there have been questions about the possibility of low progesterone in the luteal phase causing infertility, a shortened luteal phase, mid-luteal spotting, and/or miscarriage. Since progesterone is responsible for maintaining the endometrium (the lining of the uterus) and allowing implantation to occur, it stands to reason that not having enough progesterone could contribute to any or all of these phenomena. So far, however, when the scientific evidence has been examined, it has proven very difficult to specifically define luteal phase defect (LPD).

In the scientific literature, LPD has been defined inconsistently. Although it is generally accepted that a luteal phase lasting eight days or less is abnormal, the available studies have sometimes used other definitions or noted that women don't often have such consistently short luteal phases. Tests used over the years include progesterone testing (though progesterone levels in the blood fluctuate considerably throughout the day). They also include endometrial biopsy, an invasive procedure that samples the actual tissue of the uterine lining and tries to correlate its appearance (under a microscope), along with hormonal secretions, with a supposed ideal time for implantation. However, when studying LPD's possible connection to various outcomes, the available LPD tests do not conclusively predict failure to establish a healthy pregnancy, and interventions to try and improve a supposed LPD haven't been shown to consistently benefit pregnancy in natural cycles.

So, what we can conclude currently is this: If you have a concern over your luteal phase, especially if it is persistently short or you're seeing spotting, talk to your reproductive endocrinologist. There are some hormonal issues relating to thyroid or prolactin levels, for example, that certainly can inhibit proper progesterone production. Certain lifestyle factors or diagnoses (such as excessive exercise, restrictive eating, high stress, ovulation problems, recurrent miscarriages, and increasing age or decreasing ovarian reserve) may increase the risk of LPD, if such a phenomenon even exists. Given your individual circumstances, you can determine with your physician if the benefits of trying to support your luteal phase outweigh the risks. Further, you can discuss different ways of doing so, whether through supplements or other complementary approaches, progesterone suppositories, or fertility treatments to help increase your own progesterone production. But do keep in mind that, since we can't yet scientifically define LPD, these treatments are subject to the scientific opinion of your doctor; there aren't any established guidelines on the topic yet. One important action you can take on your own to try and positively impact your luteal phase is to follow a fertility-friendly lifestyle that best allows your follicle to produce the necessary progesterone.

Uterine Cycle

So far we have focused on the hormonal events of the menstrual cycle and how they drive the process of ovulation. However, ultimately, the estrogen and progesterone produced by the ovaries have to act upon the uterus to prepare for pregnancy, support early pregnancy, or to reset the uterine lining for the next cycle. Since the ovarian hormones drive the uterine actions, the phases of the ovarian and uterine cycles are intrinsically connected.

MENSTRUATION

Menstruation returns the uterine lining to its baseline state, shedding the endometrial growth from the prior cycle and returning to a single layer of endometrial cells. As described earlier, this process is generally triggered by dropping progesterone levels, which tell the body that a pregnancy was not initiated and it is now time for the uterus to reset itself for a fresh chance at pregnancy. Essentially, this signals the start of a new menstrual cycle and follicular phase. With this understanding, we can cover two caveats to menstruation.

First, not all uterine bleeding signifies that ovulation has occurred. Particularly in those women who experience infrequent periods, often accompanied by bouts of prolonged bleeding lasting weeks or months, we see something called anovulatory bleeding. In this situation, the ovarian follicles remain small, but since they are so abundant, enough estrogen is produced to allow the uterine lining, called the endometrium, to grow thicker. Even if no follicle matures and ovulates, the uterine lining grows thick enough over time that it becomes unstable and starts to break down. However, since this process does not occur through the usual pattern of progesterone exposure and withdrawal, the bleeding is often irregular and prolonged. We see this pattern frequently in polycystic ovary syndrome (discussed in chapter 2, page 16) and other situations where ovulation is not happening regularly.

Second, since menstruation is triggered by dropping progesterone levels, as long as the uterine lining was stimulated to grow by estrogen exposure and can therefore shed some tissue, the process of giving and taking away progesterone will trigger uterine bleeding, even without ovulation. Oral contraceptive pills (also discussed in chapter 2, page 29) take advantage of this mechanism; however, it is important to recognize that these bleeds are not true periods. They do not reflect ovulation.

With these caveats covered, there are certain parameters that define a normal period. Typically, it will last three to eight days, often including spotting at the beginning or end. Menstrual flow is considered abnormally heavy if it lasts longer than eight days or requires changing of menstrual products every one to two hours or more frequently. Medical attention should be sought if you are noticing these characteristics to your period.

PROLIFERATIVE PHASE

After menstruation ends, the uterus enters the proliferative phase, where the endometrium thickens in preparation for a possible pregnancy. In response to rising estrogen levels characteristic of the ovarian follicular phase, there is abundant growth of the endometrial cells. The uterine lining needs to reach a certain thickness in order to support a proper implantation, giving the placental cells enough depth to attach securely without burrowing deeper into the muscle layer of the uterus.

The process of endometrial proliferation will continue as long as estrogen is present without progesterone, which, as noted earlier, is only produced *after* ovulation. If the endometrium grows unchecked, it can eventually develop growths called endometrial polyps (which are like small skin tags growing inside the uterine cavity), endometrial hyperplasia (precancerous changes), or endometrial cancer. Thus, going long periods of time without ovulation does increase the risk of these dangerous growths (though birth control, discussed in chapter 2, can lower this risk if a progestin-including method is used). Fat tissue in our bodies can also make extra estrogen, sometimes throwing off the ovulatory cycle; therefore, being overweight adds to the risk of endometrial overgrowth.

There are a few conditions that can also cause a thin lining, the most common being scar tissue from a prior surgery or pregnancy. Chronic infections can also prevent the endometrium from reaching its full thickness, as can certain medications, which are discussed later.

SECRETORY PHASE

The secretory phase begins with the luteal secretion of progesterone, which stimulates the endometrial glands to produce substances that stabilize the lining and prevent it from starting to break down. If an egg has been fertilized in the Fallopian tube, and the resulting embryo reaches the uterine cavity, the process of implantation may begin. As the embryo burrows into the endometrium, some women will experience bleeding or cramping. It is important to recognize that such symptoms occur in the minority of women, and are not reliable indicators of pregnancy. Once implantation has progressed to where the placental precursor cells begin secreting β-hCG, not only can the pregnancy be detected first in the blood, and then by urine tests, but, as previously described, the corpus luteum is enabled to continue making progesterone and the lining remains supported.

If there is no implantation, eventually the progesterone production drops off, and the lining starts to break down. Many women will experience a day or two of spotting as this process begins, and then the full period will start. This first day of full menstrual flow marks the beginning of the next cycle.

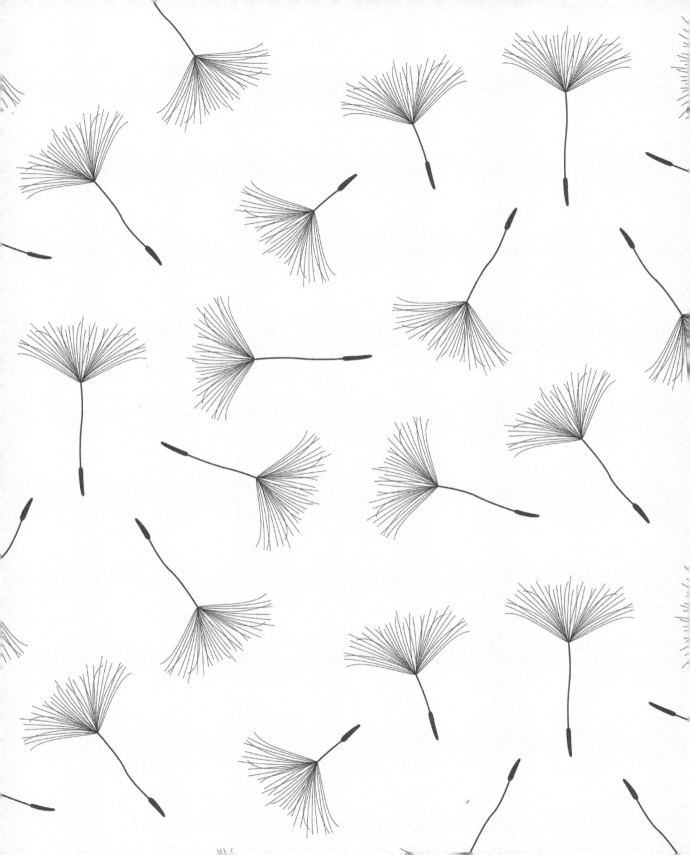

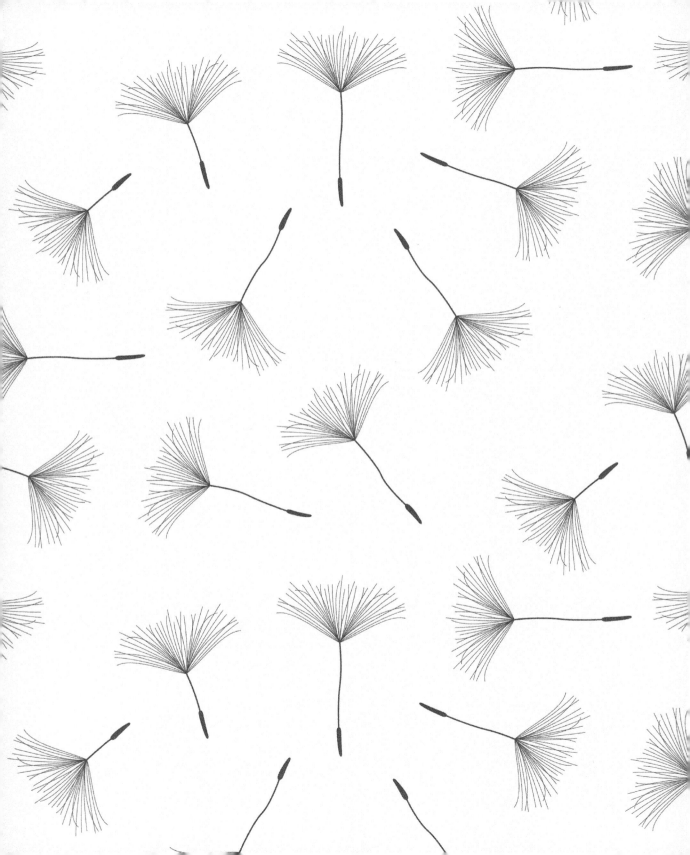

Chapter Two
Fertility Complications

Now that we have covered the basic physiology of the ovulatory menstrual cycle, let's turn our attention to some common medical conditions related to fertility. Understanding these conditions will help ensure there are no complications in your case that could influence the success of FAM, and if there are, it will help you understand how to give them further attention in order to achieve pregnancy. Though fertility is often framed as a women's issue, it is important to recognize that roughly one-third of infertility cases involve a male factor as well. We will start with a review of male factor infertility and then move through complications related to female fertility. We will discuss some of the conditions that disrupt ovulation as well as those that can impact the Fallopian tubes and uterus. These key ingredients—eggs, sperm, uterus, and tubes—are all needed for FAM to work.

All women, including those looking to conceive using donor sperm, will benefit from understanding the warning signs for different conditions. Though many women choose to pursue donor sperm insemination in the office under a physician's supervision, some start with at-home attempts; this information is equally applicable to these scenarios.

If you are concerned that any of these issues may be present, it is a good idea to discuss it with your doctor or a fertility specialist before spending more time pursuing FAM. Sometimes a diagnosis is confirmed and other times we can offer reassurance. In any case, a couple that has been trying to conceive is officially diagnosed with infertility after a year of regular unprotected intercourse if the female partner is under 35, or after six months if she is 35 years or older. Although women reach their peak fertility in their mid-20s, the likelihood of achieving pregnancy in any given month still tops out at about 25 percent. By the time they are in their early 40s, it is more like 5 to 10 percent. Statistically, then, after these lengths of trying, about 85 percent of couples will have been successful. Keep in mind that about 15 out of 100 couples—roughly one in eight—experience infertility. It is relatively common and should not be a cause of shame.

If your TTC journey has reached a length of time that meets the infertility diagnosis, it is recommended that you see a fertility specialist and undergo the basic fertility evaluation. It is worth understanding ahead of time that roughly 10 to 15 percent of couples that pursue an infertility evaluation will have all the tests come back as normal, and therefore receive a diagnosis of unexplained infertility. Though this diagnosis is very frustrating to couples, as it seems that "everything works" but they haven't yet achieved a healthy pregnancy, it is important to realize that fertility testing has limits but treatment can still be successful. Though it may feel intimidating to visit with a fertility specialist, this will truly be your best path to understanding your family-building options moving forward.

Male Infertility

The process of trying to get pregnant is often portrayed as fun, nonstop sex on television and in movies; however, this is definitely not always—or even usually—the case. Many couples struggle through the journey of trying to conceive, and partners often process their fertility journey quite differently. In general, it is ideal when both partners are on the same page regarding the desire to expand their family. However, often there are differences in how each partner experiences the process: How much are you talking about it? Do you both want to know your ovulatory status?

How much testing and treatment would you consider and in what time frame? How important is parenthood? Given the likelihood that two individuals may not answer these questions identically, it is not surprising that the process of trying to conceive quickly becomes stressful for many couples and can put a strain on the relationship.

This stress can sometimes directly impact male fertility via sexual dysfunction. Even men who are eager for fatherhood can report anxiety, loss of libido, and erectile issues. Fertility specialists see this frequently in the office, and it can quickly lead to resentment from the female partner as well as embarrassment and shame on the part of the male partner. Often the validation of how commonly this occurs is helpful to couples. Working with your physician or a therapist can help couples not only communicate better but improve the sexual dysfunction. However, it is important to recognize that sometimes this issue can be a sign of other medical problems, such as low testosterone. Therefore, it is worth a visit with a reproductive urologist to confirm, through bloodwork and a semen analysis, that there are no larger issues at play.

Despite one-third of all infertility cases relating to the male partner, it often comes as a surprise to the couple. There are known risk factors for male factor infertility, such as using anabolic steroids for bodybuilding, taking testosterone or a variety of other medications, smoking or excessive alcohol use, age, and certain medical conditions, especially cystic fibrosis or diabetes. However, men without any of these risk factors can still have fertility issues, even if they've fathered children before, so once any of these risk factors or a diagnosis of infertility has been identified, it is a good idea to get a semen analysis. A primary care provider, a urologist, or the female partner's gynecologist or fertility specialist can assist in obtaining a semen analysis. Although there are now at-home kits for semen analysis, they are not yet widely validated and should be used only as a last resort. The results can come back in four main categories: no sperm, very low motile sperm count (likely requiring in vitro fertilization, or IVF), somewhat low motile sperm count (possibly requiring intrauterine insemination, or IUI), or normal. An abnormal result should be tested again for confirmation, keeping in mind that the sperm growth cycle is about 90 days and can be impacted by serious illnesses during this time.

If there is any abnormality noted in the semen analysis, a consultation and further evaluation with a reproductive urologist can help identify hormonal, genetic, or environmental issues and treatment options. All this being said, the foundation of male fertility does share a lot with female fertility. A healthy diet, physical activity, the avoidance of toxic substances, and certain vitamins or supplements all have the potential to improve male fertility and are great, healthy choices for any man looking to become a father.

PCOS

Polycystic ovary syndrome (PCOS) is the most common hormonal disorder of reproductive-aged women. Originally called Stein-Leventhal syndrome after the doctors who recognized the pathology in the 1960s, PCOS is a multifaceted disorder with many possible manifestations, which are discussed in this section. However, one of its key features is an overlap with metabolic diseases, such as diabetes and hypertension. Though the cause of PCOS has not yet been identified, it runs strongly in families, with daughters of women with PCOS at higher risk of also having PCOS, and sons at higher risk of metabolic disease.

When it comes to diagnosing PCOS, the first step is excluding other causes of irregular menstrual cycles, such as abnormal levels of prolactin or thyroid hormones. After that, there are three sets of diagnostic criteria that can be used. The most common, the Rotterdam criteria, was released in 2003 and requires at least two out of the following three conditions to be present:

* **Irregular or absent ovulation.** As discussed earlier, a normal cycle is one that comes every 24 to 38 days, ideally with appropriately timed ovulatory and premenstrual symptoms. If the menstrual cycle falls out of this time frame, particularly if it comes in longer cycles, this is highly suggestive of irregular or absent ovulation. Aside from having ovulatory symptoms, there are a number of ways to confirm ovulation. Some of these, such as basal body temperature charting and urinary ovulation predictor kits or wearable devices, are discussed later in this book. For women under the care of a physician, other options, such as ultrasound confirmation of follicular growth or verification of progesterone levels in the bloodwork consistent with ovulation, are available.

* **Hyperandrogenism.** This criterion refers to either bloodwork results or clinical symptoms suggesting that the level of hormones like testosterone are higher than expected for the average woman. Though we often think of testosterone and other similar hormones (called androgens) as "male hormones," the reality is that women have them, too, just typically at lower levels than men. They are produced by both the ovaries and the adrenal glands, which are a pair of small hormonal organs that sit atop the kidneys and are responsible for making the primary stress hormone, cortisol.

* **Polycystic ovarian morphology.** This criterion refers to how the ovaries appear on a transvaginal ultrasound, typically with many follicles arranged on the edge of the ovary, in what is often referred to as a "string of pearls" appearance. Either the

number of follicles or the ovarian volume must exceed a threshold to qualify, and only one ovary needs to have this appearance. It is important to note that PCOS is truly a misnomer; nothing in the criteria requires having a "cyst," and the follicles seen on ultrasound are not cysts either. It is also worth knowing because these immature follicles produce anti-Müllerian hormone (AMH), which is typically elevated in women with PCOS, though this is not part of the diagnostic criteria.

PCOS Symptoms and Diagnosis

Because of the many potential impacts of PCOS, it can manifest very differently from woman to woman—and also over the course of a lifetime. Some issues may be more relevant than others during certain phases of your life, and each woman will have her own individual grouping of these possible symptoms. There is also some racial and ethnic variation in presence and severity of symptoms, especially regarding metabolic disease, hirsutism, and weight.

* **Insulin resistance.** Resistance to insulin, the hormone that processes sugar, can cause weight gain and fluctuating blood sugar levels with resultant headaches, fatigue, and more.

* **Weight gain.** Often due to insulin resistance, women with PCOS have higher rates of being overweight.

* **Hirsutism.** Hirsutism refers to extra facial or body hair, or hair in a male-pattern distribution, relative to one's ethnicity.

* **Acne.** Cystic acne can occur due to high androgen activity in the skin.

* **Thinning hair.** Also due to high androgens, male-pattern baldness or hair thinning is frequently observed.

* **Irregular bleeding.** Due primarily to anovulation, periods can come in an unpredictable fashion or not at all.

* **Pelvic pain.** Cramping during prolonged anovulatory bleeding or ovarian cysts (page 18) can cause pelvic pain.

* **Infertility.** A lack of predictable ovulation often results in infertility or difficulty getting pregnant.

* **Mood changes.** Anxiety and depression are three to five times more common in women with PCOS.

* **Sleep problems.** Higher rates of diminished sleep quality and obstructive sleep apnea have been observed.

* **Fatigue.** Fatigue can come from a variety of factors, such as mood, weight, and hormonal fluctuations, including adrenal stress hormones.

Cysts

That the name PCOS—polycystic ovary syndrome—has the word "cyst" in it remains one of the most confusing aspects of this syndrome. Some experts in the field have even recommended changing the name because having a cyst is not necessary to have PCOS. Cysts are growths in the ovary that come in many different forms, with the potential to be benign or cancerous. As described in chapter 1, in each ovulatory cycle the follicle transforms into a cyst called the corpus luteum. Since the corpus luteum is required for pregnancy to occur, this type of cyst is normal and to be expected. On the other hand, what are often described to patients as "little cysts" on an ultrasound are typically just the small ovarian follicles (fluid-filled sacs containing an immature egg)—the "string of pearls" described earlier. If stimulated properly, these follicles could actually mature and release an egg.

There are many other kinds of cysts, including some that will be discussed in the section on endometriosis (page 19). However, what is more common in women with PCOS is the presence of simple cysts—follicles that grow improperly and can get quite large, persist for months or years, and cause pain, particularly if they cause the entire ovary to twist (called an ovarian torsion) or if they rupture (sometimes bleeding heavily). These latter two possibilities, ovarian torsion and cyst rupture, often result in women requiring emergency care for severe pain and possibly surgery as well. Once a woman has had such a cyst, she is at elevated risk for having recurrent cysts. The primary method for preventing recurrence is the use of oral contraceptive pills (OCPs).

Treatment

There is no single cure that addresses every possible symptom; however, there are some lifestyle approaches that generally improve PCOS. Treatment for PCOS focuses on managing the current symptoms. A dietary approach that reduces processed, white flour products and refined carbohydrates is key, and can be combined with exercise, medication, or supplements to optimize weight and quality of life. Losing excess body weight can help normalize menstrual cycles and reduce symptoms of high androgen levels. OCPs can also assist in achieving these goals. I want to pause and validate how difficult it can be for many women with PCOS to reach their desired weight despite their best attempts. If you're struggling, or have reached a plateau, please reach out to your care team for help!

For other PCOS symptoms, additional specialized care may be necessary, for example to manage acne, hair growth, or mental health. Using OCPs also improves skin conditions, although from a mental health perspective, some women may feel their mood worsen with hormonal treatment. From a fertility perspective, the first step is preconception evaluation to look for possible health conditions, such as insulin resistance, that could increase the chance for pregnancy complications like gestational diabetes. From there, the preferred medication for ovulation induction (i.e., stimulating a follicle to grow) is letrozole, and this can be combined with intercourse as a simple intervention to help achieve pregnancy.

In summary, crafting a personalized care plan may require assembling a multidisciplinary healthcare team, possibly including a gynecologist, reproductive and/or medical endocrinologist, psychiatrist or psychologist, dermatologist, nutritionist, and/or physical trainer.

Endometriosis

Endometriosis is a condition in which the type of tissue that normally lines the inside of the uterus, called the endometrium, starts to grow in other parts of the body. Most commonly, endometriosis grows in the ovaries, or on the Fallopian tubes or other pelvic structures. There are a few theories as to how endometriosis develops. One of the most widely cited is what's known as retrograde menstruation, where menstrual blood and endometrial tissue flow backward through the tubes and attach to the pelvic structures once they exit. However, since endometriosis can spread to remote parts of the body, such as the lungs (where it can cause a bloody cough that reappears with each period), there is clearly more to the story. As with PCOS, there is a genetic component, so having a family history of endometriosis makes it more likely that you will have it as well.

The symptoms typically relate to where the endometriosis is, with the key symptom being dysmenorrhea, or incredibly painful periods. Women often report missing school or work, or experiencing diminished quality of life, due to the pain. In the following section, we cover the most common symptoms seen in women with endometriosis as well as treatment options. Fortunately, endometriosis does not typically affect one's ovulatory status; however, if the endometriosis grows into the ovaries, it can speed up the ovarian aging process and reduce ovarian reserve. Endometriosis growth can also block off the Fallopian tubes and increase inflammation, which seems to lower fertility in spontaneous cycles and even in IVF.

Endometriosis Symptoms and Diagnosis

Endometriosis tissue is hormonally active and responds to the hormonal pattern during menstruation, with worsening symptoms during that time. Based on the grouping of these symptoms, particularly the painful periods, we can make a clinical diagnosis of endometriosis. However, since many of these symptoms can be caused by a variety of other diagnoses, it can take some time for women to be diagnosed with endometriosis; this can potentially delay their treatment and compromise their fertility. If you are experiencing these symptoms, it is a good idea to speak with a gynecologist or fertility specialist. The true gold standard in diagnosis involves a minimally invasive surgery known as laparoscopy, with visual and pathologic confirmation of endometriosis tissue; this may be an appropriate choice for you. Symptoms of endometriosis include:

* **Dysmenorrhea.** Severe menstrual cramping is the most common symptom of endometriosis.

* **Dyspareunia.** Pain during intercourse can result when deep vaginal penetration results in pressure on endometriosis tissue and adjacent tender areas.

* **Pain during bowel movements.** When endometriosis implants on the intestines, it can cause pain during bowel movements, and even rectal bleeding.

* **Gastrointestinal complaints.** Diarrhea, constipation, bloating, and nausea are all frequently reported by women with endometriosis, particularly during their periods.

* **Fatigue.** Whether due to inflammation, chronic pelvic pain, or joint and nerve pain, women with endometriosis frequently report fatigue.

* **Infertility.** Endometriosis can cause scar tissue that blocks off the Fallopian tubes and/or ovarian cysts that can speed up depletion of ovarian reserve.

* **Excessive bleeding.** Women with endometriosis frequently report heavy menstrual bleeding and/or spotting in between cycles.

Scar Tissue, Adhesions, and Chocolate Cysts

As described earlier, the impacts of endometriosis are largely related to where the tissue grows. Some of the most common locations for endometriosis are throughout the pelvis, namely on the Fallopian tubes, the outside of the uterus, the ovaries, and the tissue that lines the inside of the abdomen and pelvis (called the peritoneum). Though areas of endometriosis often look like reddish burn marks, their appearance can range from clear (often in younger women) to all shades of red and brown or even white fibrous scar tissue.

The endometriosis acts like a glue, creating adhesions between structures that are not normally so tightly attached, often between the reproductive organs but also the intestines and bladder. This scar tissue can cause pain due to the abnormal adhesions as well as recurring pain during the period. It can pinch off the Fallopian tubes or encase the ovary in a web of adhesions, effectively preventing the egg from reaching the tube. These findings can be detected either by surgery or through a hysterosalpingogram (HSG), an X-ray test conducted after an injection of radiopaque dye. It is important to remember that there are other causes for blocked Fallopian tubes, especially prior pelvic infections, which can go unnoticed but can cause lasting damage, or prior pelvic surgeries resulting in internal scar tissue.

When endometriosis grows directly in the ovaries, it creates cysts full of old blood, often referred to as chocolate cysts because of the thick brownish fluid they contain. These cysts, called endometriomas, are typically detected by ultrasound or during surgery. Other imaging methods, such as CT or MRI scans, may also be able to identify endometriosis but are not as commonly used for this purpose.

Regardless of exact location, pelvic endometriosis tissue does release inflammatory factors that seem to impact egg quality. For example, in women pursuing IVF with donor eggs, if the donor had endometriosis and the recipient did not, success rates were lower than the other way around. This type of study shows that IVF can work around issues such as tubal blockages, but that there is an overall reduced fertility just by virtue of endometriosis' impact on the developing eggs. Therefore, if you have a known or suspected diagnosis of endometriosis and are trying for pregnancy, it's a good idea to seek counseling. You may also want to pursue evaluation of the tubes and ovaries. This evaluation can happen at any point along the way, but should definitely be done by the time an infertility diagnosis is reached.

Treatment

Treatment for endometriosis depends highly on the reason for intervention, namely whether the primary concern is pain, fertility, or both. The typical first-line treatment for pain involves medical approaches, and the following options can be tried in escalating fashion. Combination oral contraceptive pills (OCPs, those containing both estrogen and progesterone, reviewed on page 29) reduce activity of the endometriosis tissue, particularly when used continuously (where the placebo pills are skipped). Many women note substantially improved quality of life by avoiding the hormonal environment of menstruation, when symptoms are typically the worst. Residual pain can often be managed by nonmedical approaches, such as heating pads and rest, or with nonsteroidal anti-inflammatory drugs (NSAIDs).

If OCPs prove insufficient, stronger medications are available. These work by altering the impact of GnRH, thereby shutting down the reproductive axis. This approach is a more effective way of cutting down the hormonal exposure that causes endometriosis tissue to flare up and cause pain. However, because estrogen—whether from the ovaries or from OCPs—is necessary for bone and heart health, long-term use of these strategies requires "add-back therapy," meaning additional supplements of calcium and vitamin D to prevent osteoporosis and other complications of a low estrogen state.

The goal of medical therapy is to reduce current symptoms and prevent disease from progressing. If this approach proves unsuccessful, surgery can be considered. Surgery provides the opportunity to confirm the diagnosis and its severity as well as remove any visible endometriosis, but some caution should be used here. First, surgery is not guaranteed to improve pain, especially if the tissue is not entirely removed. Because endometriosis can grow in so many locations, this means the surgeon must be prepared for a potentially extensive resection of endometriosis off the intestines, bladder, and other tissues as well as possibly removing endometriomas as gently as possible to avoid further compromising normal ovarian tissue. Many surgeons may not feel comfortable with these complex surgeries, so it is critical to choose an experienced surgeon with special interest in this area.

When it comes to fertility, the approach is slightly different. It has been demonstrated that reflexively performing surgery on every woman with suspected endometriosis has a very low yield. There are certainly diminishing returns with repeated surgeries, as each surgery can speed up the decrease in ovarian reserve. Multiple surgeries can also increase the chances of complications such as heavy bleeding, necessitating removal of the entire ovary. However, the data is quite complex and the role of surgery is a highly individualized discussion each patient should have with their fertility specialist.

In cases where surgery has been unsuccessful or deemed unhelpful, infertility treatment, especially in vitro fertilization, which works around blocked tubes, can make the difference. Whether the endometriosis is causing tubal disease, diminished ovarian reserve, or just infertility, IVF can assist.

One final consideration is prevention: If the diagnosis is made at a relatively early stage, treatment could be undertaken to actually prevent its progression. Such options could include medical treatment—particularly birth control, not surgery—and fertility preservation via egg or embryo freezing.

Pregnancy after 35

"Geriatric," along with other comparable descriptors like "elderly" or "advanced maternal age," is a term typically applied to pregnant women aged 35 or older. These terms often relate more to billing codes rather than any judgment of a woman being "too old" to be pregnant. Indeed, looking at childbearing trends, so-called geriatric pregnancy is now incredibly common: From 1970 to 2012, the number of first births to mothers over 35 multiplied by more than nine times.

However, there is also a medical basis for marking maternal age. Though each woman is unique, and the impact of age is gradual and not tied to any particular milestone birthday, fertility begins declining by the mid-30s. Both the number of available ovarian follicles each month, known as the antral follicle count, as well as the anti-Müllerian hormone (AMH) they produce, drop. The rate of decline is thought to be most steep between the ages of 35 and 37.

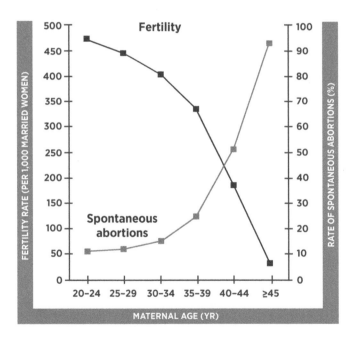

At the same time, each individual egg has an ever-increasing chance of genetic abnormalities. Therefore, the monthly pregnancy rate, about 25 percent in the mid- to late 20s, starts to drop, reaching 5 to 10 percent by age 40. Miscarriages, as well as many birth defects, are predominantly due to genetic abnormalities in the embryo or fetus, and the chances of a pregnancy loss easily approach 20 to 25 percent by the early 40s.

FERTILITY PRESERVATION

As we have discussed, our fertility declines with age primarily due to the reduced number and quality of follicles available each month. Given the reduced fertility and higher miscarriage rates that come with trying to get pregnant in the late 30s and beyond, many women and couples turn to fertility preservation. These techniques are also used by younger women who find that they have diminished ovarian reserve due to endometriosis, pelvic surgery, cancer treatment, or other reasons; by women who may be needing to start chemotherapy or radiation therapy, risking damage to the ovaries; or trans men planning to initiate or continue gender-affirming hormone treatment or pursue bottom surgery, including removal of the reproductive organs.

Fertility preservation by the freezing of either eggs or embryos (eggs that have been fertilized by sperm and have grown for five to seven days in the laboratory) is the first half of an IVF cycle, and has been a nonexperimental technique since October 2012. It involves taking injectable synthetic hormones that stimulate as many follicles as are available that month, in hopes that they will all grow together then ultimately be retrieved via an outpatient procedure, typically under intravenous sedation, and then cryopreserved. These eggs or embryos retain the chances of pregnancy associated with the age at egg retrieval rather than the age at pregnancy. It can be a very powerful tool to essentially prevent future infertility, and the grief of a difficult journey trying to conceive later in life. Talk to your gynecologist or seek consultation with a fertility specialist if you are wondering whether fertility preservation is right for you.

Thyroid Issues

The thyroid is a butterfly-shaped gland in the throat that regulates the metabolism.
The hypothalamus and pituitary gland secrete thyrotropin-releasing hormone (TRH) and thyroid-stimulating hormone (TSH), respectively, to stabilize thyroid levels. Abnormal levels of thyroid hormones are associated with menstrual irregularities, infertility, miscarriage, and birth defects.

Hypothyroidism

The pituitary compensates for low thyroid hor-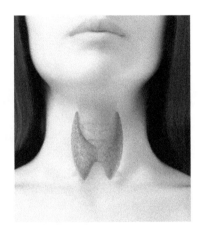mones by increasing TSH secretion, trying to nudge the thyroid into releasing sufficient amounts of hormone. With an adequate response, the diagnosis is subclinical hypothyroidism; once the thyroid cannot keep up, the individual is truly hypothyroid. Symptoms include fatigue, weight gain, feeling cold, and, often, anovulatory cycles. It is thought that the increased pituitary activity can result in not only extra secretion of TSH, but also of the other pituitary hormones, especially prolactin, but possibly FSH or LH as well. These hormonal changes disrupt the normal process of follicular recruitment and ovulation. Significant weight gain can also contribute to hormonal disruption. Anovulatory cycles are characterized by infrequent or absent periods that are nonetheless often quite heavy when they arrive.

Hyperthyroidism

When the opposite occurs and the thyroid produces too much hormone, a woman
may experience symptoms such as weight loss, palpitations, or feeling warm. The body tries to compensate with less TSH secretion, with comparable marking of subclinical (low TSH, normal thyroid hormones) and clinical hyperthyroidism (low TSH, high thyroid hormones). Through similar mechanisms of weight change and altered pituitary function, women with hyperthyroidism may stop ovulating regularly and instead see absent or light periods.

COPING WITH MISCARRIAGE

Miscarriage is one of the most common but devastating experiences a woman can undergo. Though there is no right or wrong way to emotionally react to pregnancy loss, many women do report feeling down or depressed afterward, sometimes for months or years to follow. It is so important to understand that any reaction is normal, and that if you are experiencing depression or anxiety after a loss, there are many support groups and resources that can help. It can feel stigmatizing and isolating to experience a miscarriage, and can even create strain between two partners who might both be grieving, so do not hesitate to seek help if you are struggling.

There are a few things I tell every patient I see who has experienced a miscarriage. First, pregnancy loss is extremely common. One in every four to five pregnancies ends in a miscarriage, with exponentially higher rates after age 40. The vast majority of these losses occur in the first trimester, and so each early milestone substantially lowers the risk of a loss—confirmation by ultrasound of an intrauterine pregnancy, visualization of the fetal heartbeat, beginning of the second trimester, etc. Miscarriages are most commonly caused by genetic or other anomalies that would prevent the pregnancy from being viable, and are very rarely caused by something that a woman has done. It is normal to go back and wonder if the loss happened because one exercised too intensely or ate something unusual, or any such behavior, but these activities of daily life are almost never to blame.

After one isolated miscarriage, particularly if there has been a prior healthy pregnancy, the chances remain most likely that the next pregnancy will be viable. However, once a second miscarriage has occurred, there are guidelines on certain tests that should be performed to rule out a recurring risk factor. These risk factors can include uterine issues like fibroids or endometrial polyps, autoimmune and blood clotting conditions, hormonal issues (especially relating to thyroid hormone), and genetic abnormalities. Each of these has a treatment that can reduce the risk to a future pregnancy. There are many tests available that fall outside of these recommendations, and it is worth discussing with your gynecologist or fertility specialist which guidelines are the basis for your evaluation.

Jessica was a 36-year-old who came to see me after two miscarriages. She had no idea what could have caused her losses and had waited more than a year after the most recent loss to seek care because she was traumatized by the experience and afraid to try again. She had even gone back on contraception to avoid the possibility of another pregnancy. In our initial consultation, we performed a vaginal ultrasound and saw a large endometrial polyp sitting in the uterus. We scheduled an outpatient surgical procedure to remove the polyp within a few weeks. Jessica decided to come back off the birth control, and two months later she achieved a healthy pregnancy.

I have seen many other relatively straightforward fixes, for example, women with undiagnosed hypothyroidism who normalized their hormone levels with medication and then conceived. However, often no explanation is uncovered or more treatment seems required, in which case the approach is highly individualized and based on the priorities of the woman or couple. I have seen many patients like Flora, a 41-year-old who had a history of three very early losses over the previous two years. One of these was a biochemical pregnancy, where the miscarriage occurs so early that the pregnancy is not even visible on ultrasound. The other two had happened by five to six weeks. Though it can be possible to test pregnancy tissue for its genetic status, she had all the miscarriages at home and did not have any such testing. Neither her nor her partner's evaluations were unusual. We determined that age and the associated risk of genetic abnormalities was likely the issue, and she decided to move on to in vitro fertilization treatment, with preimplantation testing of the embryos. Once we got to the point of an embryo transfer of a normal embryo, she was successful on the first try and continued on with a healthy pregnancy. There are many ways to reach your success story after miscarriage, so don't lose hope and do seek expert help if you're struggling.

The Pill and Your Cycle

Hormonal birth control functions by supplying the body with components that typi-cally resemble both ovarian hormones, estrogen and progesterone. The presence of these hormones signals to the pituitary gland that further secretion of FSH and LH hormone is unnecessary, so follicular growth and ovulation are typically prevented. The estrogen component most effectively suppresses follicular growth, and the progesterone-like or progestin component produces an endometrium and cervical mucus that are unfavorable to pregnancy. Some options that include both estrogen and a progestin are the combined oral contraceptive pill, the patch, and the ring.

Some approaches only contain the progestin component. These are most useful for women who cannot take estrogen-containing contraception, either for medical reasons or because they are breastfeeding or smoke tobacco. These options include the progesterone-only "minipill," progesterone-containing intrauterine devices (IUDs) or implantable devices, and the injectable depot medroxyprogesterone acetate (Depo-Provera).

There are also nonhormonal options, such as the copper IUD, spermicides, barrier methods, and fertility awareness or calendaring methods. Aside from the copper IUD, hormonal options are generally more effective when studied in typical use, and offer many additional benefits, including controlling and reducing menses and its associated symptoms, preventing progression of endometriosis, ovarian cysts, and possibly fibroids, in addition to reducing the risk of endometrial, ovarian, and colorectal cancers. However, many women prefer nonhormonal methods, particularly if they track their cycles or experience side effects from hormonal options, and can consider these alternatives as appropriate.

Regarding fertility, it is important to recognize that hormonal contraception does not impair fertility, nor does it prevent the effect of age on ovarian reserve and egg quality. Even when using a method that prevents ovulation, groups of follicles still start the process of growing and atrophying, and are therefore still lost each month. Studies indicate that, with the current low-dose formations, even though it can sometimes take a few months for a menstrual cycle to return to its internally driven pattern after long-term OCP use, by one to two years after pill discontinuation pregnancy rates are not impacted by contraception use.

With hormonal contraception, the main fertility consideration is that, by preventing the body from regulating the menstrual cycle itself, ongoing changes can be masked. I have seen many patients over the years who found that after years or decades of long-term contraceptive use, their cycle is different than what they remembered—typically due to age or changes in weight or health. Therefore, many women on hormonal contraception looking to conceive in the near future may consider switching to a nonhormonal alternative for a few months, and begin tracking their menstrual cycle so as to reacquaint themselves with their current pattern.

Oral Contraceptives

Available in combined (estrogen and progestin) and progesterone-only versions, oral contraceptive pills (OCPs) come in a wide variety of options. Combined pills typically include 21 to 24 days of active, hormone-containing pills with three to seven inert placebo pills, during which the period will occur. Though some formulations include a gradually increasing estrogen dose (triphasic), most are monophasic, with a constant estrogen dose throughout the active pills. Certain pills come in an extended form, where active pills will continue for 12 weeks prior to a scheduled period, allowing the user to only experience four periods a year. There is also a wide variation in the progestin component used in formulating different pills, and due to this and other differences between pills, some women find themselves feeling better with one versus another. Sometimes experimentation is required to find the best match for each person.

Patches

Less commonly used than the pill but similar in concept as an estrogen-progestin option, the patch is applied once each week and replaced with a new patch each subsequent week for three weeks, followed by a patch-free week when the period is expected. The side effects are similar to OCPs, but some women also experience skin irritation or discoloration. There is also a higher rate of breast discomfort in the first few months. As with pills, skipping the patch-free week would allow for the spacing out of periods.

Ring

The final estrogen-progestin option is the contraceptive ring. Typically, the flexible ring is placed in the vagina for three weeks and then removed for a week, when the period will occur. Like the pills and patch, the ring-free week can be skipped, allowing for less frequent periods. Typically, a new ring is placed for the next cycle, but the newest brand of contraceptive ring can be reused for up to a year.

Shot (Depo-Provera)

Depot medroxyprogesterone acetate (formulated under the brand name Depo-Provera) is an injectable form of progestin-only contraception that is given every three months. It is a highly effective contraceptive option that strongly suppresses the menstrual cycle. As a result, however, it may cause the longest return to natural cycling, with a delay to conception of about nine months after the last injection. Further, because it is non-estrogen-containing and still prevents ovulation, it is the sole progestin-only method that increases the risk of bone loss and osteoporosis. For this reason, women generally are counseled regarding supplemental ways to protect their bone health, and the U.S. Food and Drug Administration (FDA) suggests that women should not use this contraceptive for more than two years continuously.

LARCS

Intrauterine devices (IUDs) are one of the long-acting reversible contraceptives (LARCs). Aside from Paragard, the copper-containing IUD, the others all contain a progestin component and are approved for three to five years of use. IUDs are placed by a gynecologist or other healthcare provider in the office and can be used by all women, including immediately after delivering a baby. Based on their size, some IUDs are geared specifically toward those who have never had a vaginal birth, though these typically last for a shorter period of time. Progestin-containing IUDs have many other potential benefits, including reducing the amount of menstrual bleeding and pain, treatment of endometriosis and fibroids, and protection against benign and malignant endometrial growths.

The current implantable inserts are the other category of LARC, and consist of a small, progestin-containing rod that is inserted under the skin in the upper arm. Implants are approved for use for three years, at which point a new one can be inserted. Implants can similarly reduce menstrual bleeding and pain, and provide some relief from endometriosis pain. Both types of LARCs can cause irregular bleeding, especially in the first few months after insertion.

Case Study: FAM to the Rescue

Over the years, I have taken care of many patients for whom the education and test-ing in our initial infertility evaluation was enough to help them reach their goal. After months or years of unsuccessfully trying to conceive, learning how to recognize the body's signals can sometimes be enough to make the difference. This is most true for the women who are unsure about their ovulatory status.

For example, Shivani was a 38-year-old who had gotten married about a year before meeting with me. By that point, she had been off of hormonal contraceptives for four months, after having been on them since her teen years. She was concerned that her menstrual cycle came every 24 to 25 days, and that this was shorter than what she thought she remembered about her cycle before pills. Her bleeding was also heavier than it had ever been on pills, and she was unsure if this was significant or not. She elected to complete a basic infertility evaluation. In our conversation, we were able to review a few key points.

First, as ovaries age, typically in the late 30s and early 40s, the first sign of diminish-ing ovarian reserve is a menstrual cycle that gets shorter in length, for example going from every 27 to 28 days to a pattern like Shivani's, resulting in an earlier ovulation (in this case, around cycle day 10 or 11). We measured her follicle count by ultrasound and her AMH level, and confirmed that her ovarian reserve was appropriate for her age. Second, we discussed the difference between withdrawal bleeds on birth control and true periods, and that her bleeding pattern was actually normal. We were also able to confirm via ultrasound and hysterosalpingogram (HSG) that her uterus looked normal. Finally, we discussed the natural fertility rates in this age group, likely a 10 to 15 percent chance of pregnancy each month, and that she would be considered infertile if she reached a full six months of trying without success.

After all this, we reviewed her options. She said that she would have considered IVF to allow for preservation of extra embryos for future use, but that she and her husband planned for only one child, so they would try on their own for a few more months and then gradually incorporate treatment as needed. However, none of this was needed because once she had learned to look out for signs of ovulation earlier in her cycle and time intercourse to her symptoms, she conceived two months later.

Similarly, Monique had also noticed changes in her cycle. She had PCOS but had conceived twice before on her own by making changes to her diet. Both pregnancies had been complicated by gestational diabetes, and she had gained 50 pounds from her weight prior to the first pregnancy. Once she had her IUD removed to try for her third child at age 33, she was surprised to find that her cycle had gone from every 34 days to every 50 to 65 days. We completed an evaluation similar to Shivani's, and identified that with this weight gain and PCOS history Monique was no longer ovulating. Her screening tests also indicated she was prediabetic. Concerned by this information, we created a specialized diet and exercise plan, combined with metformin and supplements, with the aim of losing some of her baby weight. Within four months she had lost nearly 30 pounds and had moved her sugar levels back into a healthy range. During this time, her menstrual cycle started to return to her prior pattern, and she could again recognize ovulatory changes to her cervical mucus. By the sixth month, she was pregnant. Even better, since she began her pregnancy understanding her diagnosis and metabolic risks, she was able to continue her healthy lifestyle, which prevented her from developing gestational diabetes for a third time.

Though many cases of irregular periods or infertility require more intervention than these women did, both were able to utilize FAM to understand and adapt to their changing menstrual patterns and grow their families as a result.

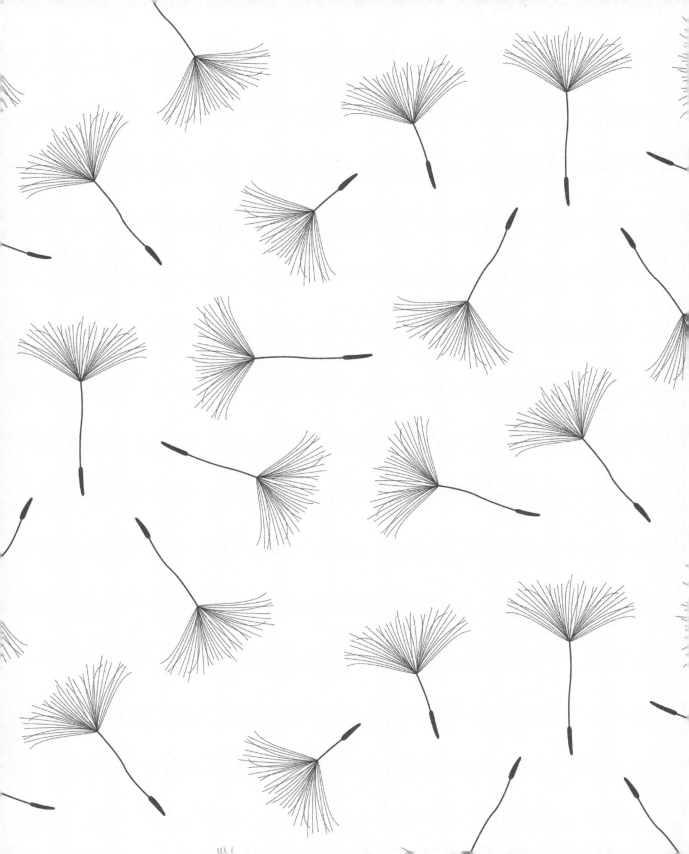

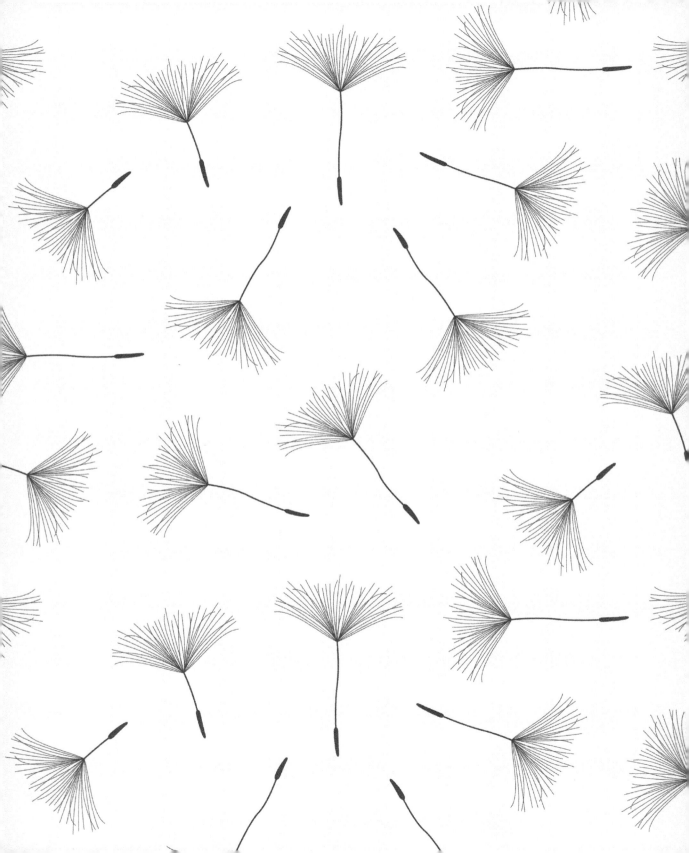

Chapter Three

Fertility Awareness Methods Explained

In this chapter, we will cover the history behind the fertility awareness method (FAM), setting the stage for the chapters that follow, where we will dive into the nitty-gritty details. In discussing these methods, you'll quickly see that FAM is actually an umbrella term encompassing a variety of techniques that can track ovulation. These techniques can be used individually or in combination with one another to pinpoint the fertile window. There are advantages and disadvantages to each.

Regardless of method, the shared central goal of FAM is identification of the fertile window. In theory, figuring out the six fertile days in each cycle can be used to time intercourse with the goal of achieving or avoiding pregnancy. The approach in this book will help you quickly identify if you need additional evaluation or alternate interventions, and we will focus on FAM as a method of fertility promotion, not contraception. Although it is likely true that a woman who has extremely regular cycles and uses a more comprehensive FAM technique is achieving high-efficiency contraception, the data in published studies and the real-life numbers of all women who rely on FAM are less reassuring.

I only recommend FAM for contraception in those women who would not be entirely opposed to a pregnancy. I take care of women in this situation frequently—they may come in to learn more about their fertility with the intention to start a family soon, so an early positive would be just fine. For women for whom pregnancy is strictly undesired or unsafe, there are many better options.

What Is FAM?

By now you must be ready to learn everything about FAM. Understanding the key steps of the menstrual cycle was the first step because these events, and the hormonal patterns accompanying them, create the typical signs and symptoms that constitute FAM. By looking out for these signs, women can create a chart that plots out their fertile and nonfertile days, with increasing accuracy as time goes on.

Let's briefly review the biology discussed in chapter 1: As women approach ovulation, the growing follicle secretes increasing amounts of estrogen, finally triggering a spike in the luteinizing hormone (LH) that causes ovulation to occur. The follicle releases the mature egg inside, after which time it switches primarily from estrogen to progesterone production. Being sensitive to the signs of rising estrogen helps identify impending ovulation, and signs of progesterone production confirm it. Recognizing and charting these signs is what FAM is all about.

In order to identify your fertile window, the signs of rising estrogen are most important. These indicate ovulation, which signals the most important days for intercourse. The primary sign of rising estrogen is the progressive change of cervical fluid, or cervical mucus, and cervical position. Chapter 4 will discuss how to monitor the cervix. (Saliva ferning, a less popular method for detecting a rise in estrogen, which involves observing saliva samples under a microscope at home, is discussed in chapter 8, page 123.)

After ovulation, the estrogen level drops rapidly, and the signs described earlier disappear. In their place, the elevation in progesterone causes the core body temperature to rise by 0.5 to 1 degree Fahrenheit. Tracking this shift, known as basal body temperature charting, can confirm ovulation. Consistent tracking over time can help identify the typical timing of ovulation within your cycle. For a small subset of women, the temperature dips on the day of ovulation, but by and large basal body temperature charting can be most helpful in confirming the pattern hinted at by the signs of rising estrogen. If the temperature stays elevated or rises further beyond the expected duration of the luteal phase, it may even provide a tip-off to a positive pregnancy test.

In summary, by charting some or all of these signs, we can identify our fertile window. This method works most smoothly and easily for those women who have regular cycles and are willing to input more data consistently. The more certain a woman is about her fertile window, the more she can specifically time intercourse and reap the benefits of FAM, making the effort of tracking these ovulatory signs and symptoms most worthwhile. On the other hand, I have had many patients frustrated by conflicting or unclear signs in their FAM charts. I believe strongly that if using FAM is giving you extra anxiety, it is time to seek professional help. There are many ways your fertility specialist can help monitor and clarify your cycle if the methods described here present a confusing picture.

Transitioning from HBC to FAM

Many women interested in FAM are either planning to or have recently discontinued a form of hormonal birth control (HBC). As discussed in chapter 2, HBC provides the body with ovarian hormones, typically both progesterone and estrogen, resulting in suppression of the body's innate drive to ovulate. The withdrawal bleeds one might get in between pill packs or contraceptive ring insertions do not reflect hormonal patterns. Therefore, it is not useful to practice FAM while on HBC, as we would not expect to see ovulatory shifts. Even in the case of an accidental ovulation, which happens most commonly when pills are missed, the typical signs may well be muted by the contraceptive.

The only exception might be for women who are on the progesterone-only minipill while lactating. Breastfeeding releases hormones that prevent ovulation and keep estrogen and progesterone levels low. However, as one starts the weaning process, ovulation will eventually resume, with the first ovulation preceding the first period. Therefore, paying attention to the return of fertile cervical fluid may well be the first hint that your ovulatory pattern is returning. It is helpful to know that other women use progesterone-only methods because estrogen is medically unsafe for them. These women typically have the most at stake in the case of an unplanned pregnancy, and FAM alone should not be the contraceptive plan in this situation.

All that said, patients may ask when they should transition off of HBC in preparation for trying to conceive. There is no universal answer; every woman is different. Aside from progesterone injections, which suppress innate ovulatory drive the longest, ovulation can resume within weeks of HBC discontinuation with the most common types of HBC.

There are two sensible approaches to this transition. The first and most straightforward option is simply not to come off until you are definitely ready to be pregnant. However, because many women want to start tracking their cycle and reacquainting themselves with their hormonal patterns in preparation, the second option is to stop using HBC and switch to nonhormonal barrier methods, such as condoms, until ready to conceive. Many women choose the second option because they are concerned about post-pill amenorrhea, which is an extended (six months or more) lack of spontaneous ovulation in menstruation. Fortunately, the available data indicate the actual prevalence of post-pill amenorrhea is low, around 1 percent.

Women on long-term HBC, particularly if they started in their teen years, also may not know they've had an ovulatory issue, and so fertility-complicating diagnoses are only discovered after getting off HBC. The decision about how to manage your transition should be guided by your history, the type of HBC you've been utilizing and for how long, any suspicion of ovulatory or fertility diagnoses, and your family-building plan. You can always work with a gynecologist or fertility specialist if you need guidance.

THE HISTORY OF FAM

The scientific knowledge about cycles and signs that are at the core of fertility awareness methods (FAM) are largely discoveries of the 20th century. Ancient texts are rife with misunderstandings about fertility. Though some preliminary observations regarding cyclic changes in temperature and cervical fluid were made in the 1800s, it wasn't until the early 1900s when a Dutch gynecologist, Theodoor Hendrik Van de Velde, connected the biphasic (two-phase) temperature pattern to ovulation. In the 1920s, gynecologists Kyusaku Ogino in Japan and Hermann Knaus in Austria independently identified that ovulation occurs about 14 days prior to the next period. Ogino used this information to try to assist infertile couples, feeling that the failure rate of this method for contraception was unacceptably high. Nonetheless, this type of calendaring contraceptive method eventually became known as the Knaus-Ogino method.

In the Netherlands, Johannes Smulders, a Roman Catholic physician, utilized this information to more formally develop a calendar-based contraceptive method. Working with the Dutch Roman Catholic medical association to promote these teachings, his work became the foundation of the rhythm method promoted by the Catholic Church for decades to come. In the 1930s, Catholic physicians across the world spread these teachings, including pioneering US gynecologist John Rock, who established the first US rhythm clinic to teach FAM to Catholic couples. Once Wilhelm Hillebrand, a German Catholic priest, incorporated basal body temperature into the method, and John Billings established the connection between cervical fluid and ovulation in the 1960s, the foundations of knowledge necessary for accurate FAM practices were laid.

In the era that followed, many FAM movements proliferated. The Creighton Model, also referred to as NaPro (natural procreative) Technology, modified the Billings Ovulation Method (BOM) into a formalized instructional format. Various religious universities offered their own unique approaches, such as the Standard Days Method (SDM) from the Institute for Reproductive Health at Georgetown University, and the Marquette Method from the Institute for Natural Family Planning at Marquette University. Some of these methods are covered in more detail in chapters to come.

Importantly, in the 1980s, the FAM movement also transitioned beyond the religious realm. The first-generation proponents of secular FAM utilization included Barbara Feldman, who founded the Fertility Awareness Center in 1981, and Toni Weschler, whose book *Taking Charge of Your Fertility*, first published in 1995, immensely raised the profile of FAM among non-Catholics. Thus, broad access to FAM teachings is still relatively new, and many women are still unaware of these options. Ultimately, women deserve all the information available about their bodies, and many will choose to combine elements of both FAM and Western medical traditions as they build their families.

FAM Pros and Cons

As a method of promoting awareness of your reproductive health and fertility, FAM offers some pros and cons. Let's see how they stack up. Remember, if you find the cons outweighing the pros for you, it may indicate that seeking expert help is in order. If you're struggling with your charting, don't stress, and don't suffer alone in silence.

PROS:

* **Increased understanding of your body.** Having an awareness of what is happening in your body, and how your cycle may influence how you feel physically and mentally, is empowering.

* **Awareness of possible reproductive health issues.** The menstrual cycle is your body's fifth vital sign. FAM charting can help identify potential problems or hormonal imbalances that need expert attention.

* **Identification of the fertile window.** Most women who ovulate and use a thorough FAM method will be able to pinpoint their fertile window and time intercourse accordingly, maximizing chances of pregnancy.

* **Sexual benefits.** When following their cycles, many women notice an enhanced libido around ovulation.

* **A collaborative opportunity.** Some couples thrive on the ability to understand the different phases of one's cycle, knowing when chances of pregnancy are highest.

* **Inexpensive option.** Compared to random intercourse, FAM can make the process of trying for pregnancy more precise without much cost or any in-office care.

* **No side effects.** With no medications in the mix, there are no side effects of FAM, and no impact on any medications that you take.

CONS:

* **Effort.** FAM could be considered a lifestyle. Accurate charting typically requires daily temperature checks first thing in the morning and awareness and tracking of other signs. For some women, particularly if they struggle with infertility, these efforts can become stressful, disheartening, and burdensome.

* **Impractical for some.** For women whose lives include regular travel or certain medications, FAM may not be able to pinpoint ovulation, even if it's happening.

* **Inconsistent for some.** For women whose ovulation is absent or irregular, FAM may prove frustrating or anxiety-provoking.

* **Time.** Charting your fertile signs is not a one-and-done. It takes a few cycles of tracking before you can feel confident identifying a pattern.

* **Stressful sex.** For some couples, identifying the most fertile time creates a lot of anxiety. Some men find a sudden onset of erectile dysfunction, and women often feel resentful if intercourse is missed after the hard work expended in tracking.

* **Contraceptive limitations.** As a contraceptive, FAM has a typical-use failure rate that is unacceptable to many couples and does not offer prevention from sexually transmitted infections.

Is FAM Right for Me?

When it comes to reproductive health and fertility awareness, women are often on a spectrum. On one end are women who want to actively manage and track their bodily functions. They plan their lives around their cycle, adjusting activity levels, diet, and personal or professional commitments as needed. On the other end are those frustrated by their cyclic changes, especially if they suffer from pain, heavy bleeding, or an unpredictable cycle. They're looking for some stability. In the middle might be women who want to be highly bodily aware, but find it difficult to adhere to the daily monitoring requirements of FAM, or whose lifestyle—through frequent travel, night-shift work or an otherwise irregular schedule, certain medications, etc.—makes it difficult.

No one perspective is better than another. What matters most is knowing yourself and being realistic about whether FAM will help you feel empowered or frustrated. Improper use of FAM is certainly associated with unintended pregnancies in those who attempt to use it for contraception, but for those trying for pregnancy, it often results in a delay in seeking fertility care. I have cared for many women who spent years chasing perfect charts, only to belatedly recognize the signs that it is time for outside help.

Here is a patient that demonstrates the point. Alicia was a busy 34-year-old mother of an active four-year-old. She had conceived her daughter easily, gaining only 19 pounds during the pregnancy. She stayed home with her daughter for two years before returning to part-time work. Intense studio fitness classes were her stress management and me-time go-to, and she was 15 pounds under her prepregnancy weight. Although she desperately wanted to expand her family, since becoming a mother her libido had diminished. She had used a progesterone-releasing IUD for contraception after the delivery, but it had been removed 18 months prior, and, though she never tracked her cycles, she thought they seemed more irregular and lighter than before the pregnancy, perhaps even skipping some months.

We reviewed basic reproductive biology and how to track cycles as well as the connection between weight and cycle regularity. Alicia's bloodwork showed that she was on the verge of hypothalamic amenorrhea, when the hypothalamus in the brain shuts down the reproductive axis, in this case likely due to extreme exercise, stress, and fatigue—a finding that motivated her to make some changes. We strategized some simple methods to improve diet and incorporate some gentler exercise, mental health self-care, and personal time every week. Within a few months, she was feeling less stressed and had gained some weight, getting back to a normal body mass index. In the two months after that, she noted a period coming every 30 days with clear signs of ovulation around day 16. On the third regular cycle, she conceived a healthy pregnancy.

As this case demonstrates, utilization of FAM could have helped Alicia realize that she needed help a year or more before we actually met. She had believed that eating lightly with vigorous workouts was healthy, but once she learned what was going on with her cycle and what her body was trying to tell her, she decided to commit to the FAM lifestyle and to create a healthier environment in her household, from which her daughter and husband also benefited. Given her young age and prior successful delivery, she was a good candidate for these natural methods of optimizing and monitoring her fertility, and a great example of how FAM can work.

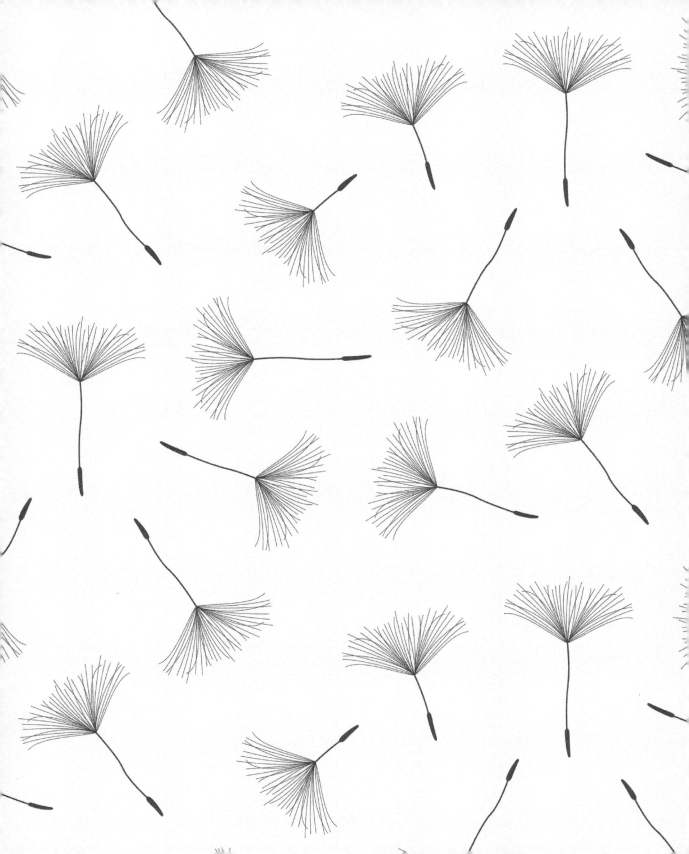

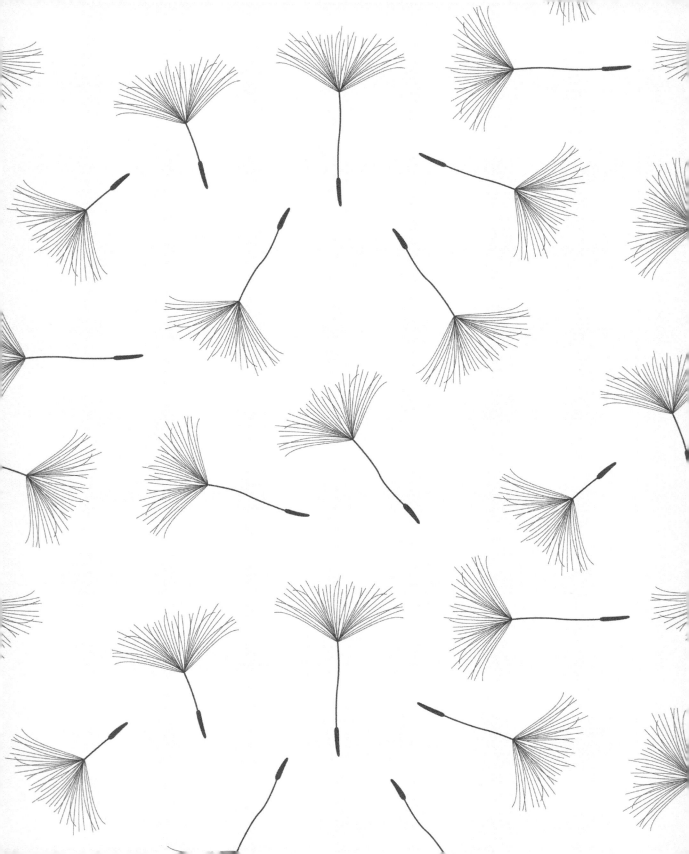

Chapter Four
Calendar Methods

In this chapter, we will examine calendar methods of fertility awareness. These options are simple: All they require is tracking the dates of your period and using that knowledge to estimate the fertile window. Though this makes them quite easy to follow, it also means that these methods require months of observing your individual pattern before you can draw accurate inferences. This extended tracking allows you to pick up and account for the variability from one cycle to the next. These methods can also result in less precision in any given cycle because they are derived from prior data, not from any prospective information in that cycle itself.

Anyone who has used fertility apps, which are discussed in chapter 8, will be familiar with the concept of monitoring past cycles to generate information about the upcoming fertile window. However, when cycle dates are the only information, apps can only average the prior data to identify a five- to six-day fertile window. The calendar method is somewhat broader in that it focuses on the outliers to generate a wider window that should not miss the most fertile days but may be quite imprecise for any given cycle.

Calendar methods are most useful to women who have consistent cycles. The more variability, the more imprecise the timing. However, they are an improvement on the misconception many women have that just aiming for the middle of one's cycle, or for day 14, is the most effective. The process of tracking your periods can also help you learn a few key facts about your cycle. Later chapters will discuss additional signs that can be added to this method to help improve precision.

What Is the Calendar Method?

Calendar methods, also referred to as the rhythm method, revolve around monitoring the dates of the menstrual cycle to identify the fertile window. As we have discussed previously, the follicular phase—or the time from period to ovulation—can vary substantially not only from woman to woman, but sometimes from cycle to cycle in the same woman. Still, cycle tracking is the basic first step to all FAM methods. By watching the length of menstrual cycles over time, you can understand how regular your cycle is, and eventually determine how precise of a fertile window you can identify by dates alone.

Though you could start trying to determine your fertile window once you've completed the first month of cycle tracking, unless that cycle happens to represent your consistent pattern, you will get more reliable results once you have several months of data to analyze. Therefore, using this method when you are actively ready to conceive can be frustrating. I do highly recommend this method, though, for women transitioning off of hormonal birth control. As discussed in chapter 2, depending on the method of contraception you were using and how strong your internal ovulatory drive is, it can take a few months for your cycle to settle back into its pattern once the impact of external hormones fades away. As you start thinking about growing your family, tracking cycles and identifying your fertile window is an important first step. During this transition off of hormonal contraception, you can use barrier methods to prevent pregnancy until you are ready to conceive.

The Steps of the Calendar Method

The calendar method is based on the reality that it is only the minority of women who have a textbook pattern of ovulating on day 14 of a 28-day cycle. So, the steps to calendar charting all revolve around tracking your dates and then calculating the possible fertile window for upcoming cycles. The longer you track, and the more data you incorporate into your assessment, the more likely you are to correctly identify your fertile window.

As you collect this data, keep an eye on the cycle lengths you're observing. The first day of full-flow bleeding is cycle day one. You can track any spotting that you may get leading up to your period or in mid-cycle, but you are focusing on the first day of a period that should feel fairly similar from month to month in terms of the amount and length of bleeding as well as associated symptoms.

If your cycle lengths seem not to fall within the normal range of every 24 to 38 days, stop and seek medical evaluation. Having an abnormally short or long cycle can signal that you're not ovulating or suggest other relevant fertility issues that you'll want to know about sooner rather than later.

STEP 1: RECORD THE CYCLES

Step one is simple but important—tracking the onset of your period. You'll count the first day of full-flow bleeding as cycle day one, and note this date on a paper calendar, planner, or app. All that is required for this step is tracking your day one dates.

Once you chart more than one start date, count the days between these cycle starts to calculate the length of the cycle. For some women it's like clockwork, with a consistent cycle length each month; others will experience substantial variation. Of course, there is no way to know in which category you fall until you've been tracking for at least a few months.

In general, it is recommended that you track for at least six months. To illustrate how this method works, imagine that you have tracked for six months and have calculated the following cycle lengths: 26, 24, 28, 27, 29, and 26 days, respectively. These numbers can be used to move on to the next step.

STEP 2: FIND THE SHORTEST CYCLE

The second step is to identify your shortest cycle. In this example, the second month was the shortest, at 24 days. We then subtract 18 from this number to determine the first fertile day. To understand why, remember that in the menstrual cycle the fertile window includes the day of ovulation and the four to five days preceding it. The luteal phase, from ovulation to the next period, typically lasts 13 to 14 days. So, by taking the entire cycle length and subtracting 18, we work backward to get that cycle's earliest fertile day. In this example of a 24-day cycle, that earliest fertile day would be cycle day six.

Some women experience persistently short cycles with a full week or more of menstrual bleeding. If your fertile window is falling during your period, you should seek evaluation. As you can imagine, the uterine lining remains unprepared for implantation while the period is ongoing, so this timing can present fertility issues.

STEP 3: FIND THE LONGEST CYCLE

Next, find your longest cycle. In this example, the fifth month tracked was a 29-day cycle. You would then subtract 11, accounting for a potentially short luteal phase, to identify the last fertile day of the cycle. In this case, subtracting 11 from 29 would give us cycle day 18.

If you begin to suspect a persistently short luteal phase lasting less than 12 days, it is also worth seeking evaluation for any further tests or treatment.

STEP 4: ESTABLISH THE FERTILITY WINDOW

Finally, you can establish the fertile window. In this example, it is quite long—from days six to 18. As you can see, despite the fertile window being only six days long in any given cycle, the relatively high cycle-to-cycle variability in this example results in 13 days being included.

In other words, the calendar method in this case suggests a potential fertile time frame of nearly two weeks, though for each individual cycle, less than half of those days will truly be part of the fertile window.

As you can see from the example, this method assumes that *any* cycle could be as short as your shortest prior cycle, or as long as your longest prior cycle, which creates a larger fertile window. During this fertile window couples trying to conceive should aim for intercourse at least every other day. There is not a significant improvement in success rates with increasing coital frequency to every day, so do not feel pressured to do so.

The Standard Days Method

If you find that your cycle length is consistently in the 26- to 32-day range, then you can utilize the Standard Days Method (SDM). It uses calculations similar to those used earlier in the calendar method example and assigns cycle days 8 to 19 as the fixed fertile window. This method is really only useful for women who are familiar with their pattern and feel confident that they cycle with that 26- to 32-day length. Typically, more than one cycle a year outside of that range indicates that this method is not advisable because the fertile window can fall outside the fixed range.

Women who choose the Standard Days Method use either an app or a beaded bracelet, called CycleBeads, to help them track their fertile or nonfertile days. The CycleBeads bracelet has 32 beads to track the days in each cycle. The first bead is red to signify the first day of the period. Adjacent to this red bead is a black cylinder with an arrow showing the direction in which the bracelet is oriented. Each morning, a rubber ring is moved to the next bead in the bracelet. Days two to seven, as well as days 20 to 32, are brown nonfertile beads, and days 8 to 19 are white beads representing the fertile window for intercourse.

There is a dark brown bead that points out day 26, to help alert you if your cycle is not reaching that minimum length necessary for this method to work. If you reach the 32nd bead without the next period starting and are not pregnant, then similarly the cycle is too long for this method.

Problems with the Calendar and Standard Days Methods

Calendar methods are simple and low-tech; however, they do present substantial shortcomings. Women with short or long cycles cannot use Standard Days. Even with the more general calendar method, women with variable cycle lengths may find their calculated fertile window is too long to be useful.

However, even for women who do ovulate and have cycle lengths within the normal range, the calculated fertile window can last from eight days to two weeks. Even with intercourse every other day, this creates four to five or more mandated intercourse nights per cycle. I routinely see couples seeking care because they are having difficulty maintaining this coital frequency due to stress or anxiety, jobs that require traveling, or any number of other considerations. As a result, many women turn to the methods discussed in the upcoming chapters to further fine-tune the prediction of ovulation timing, narrow down the fertile window, and more precisely time intercourse.

There are a few other considerations with a calendar method. First, tracking your cycle day one dates accurately is extremely important. Being off by a day or two can impact your calculations. Further, because this method is historical, if you experience a cycle that is shorter or longer than any previously recorded cycle, the calculations will be inaccurate. Stress or illness are among the most frequent causes for such unanticipated changes. If there is such an explanation for an aberrant cycle, you could exclude it from future calculations. However, if there's no clear explanation, the fertile window should be recalculated, taking the irregular cycle into account.

All of this said, the sole impact of an unexpectedly irregular cycle or inaccurate calculations is that some or all of the fertile window may be missed. Those women or couples who are either further along in the process of trying to conceive, or who truly wish to maximize their chances each month and reduce the chances of missing the fertile window, would benefit from some of the methods discussed next.

Given this discussion, you might see quite clearly why using a calendar method alone for contraception is not at all advisable. Its imprecision could result in abstinence being required for almost half the month, which is likely not desirable for most couples. Further, if at any time a cycle is shorter or longer than those previously tracked, there may be fertile days outside of the calculated window. Though this book is focused on FAM methods for conceiving rather than avoiding pregnancy, it is important that calendaring be combined with other methods to even be considered a medically advisable contraceptive option.

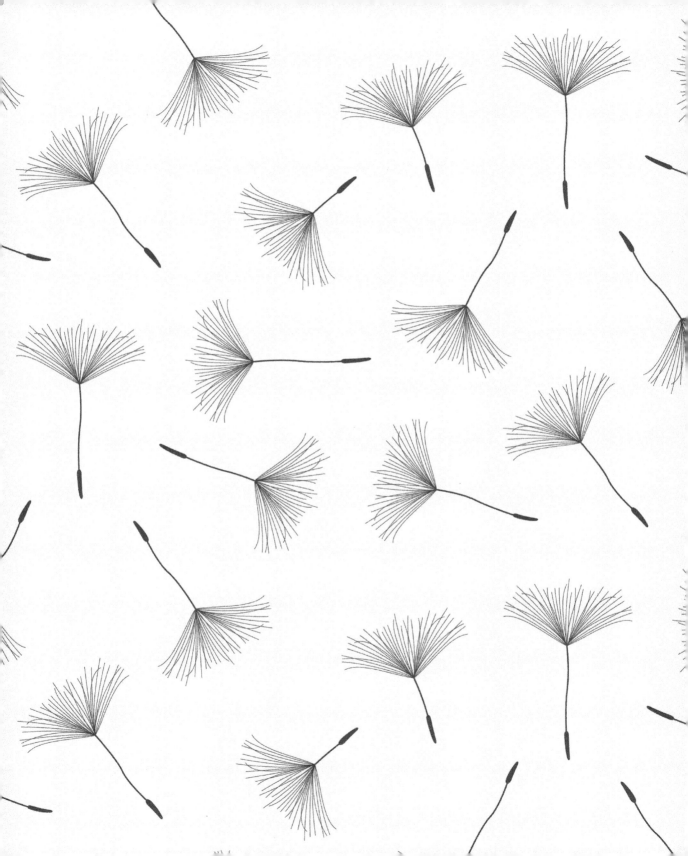

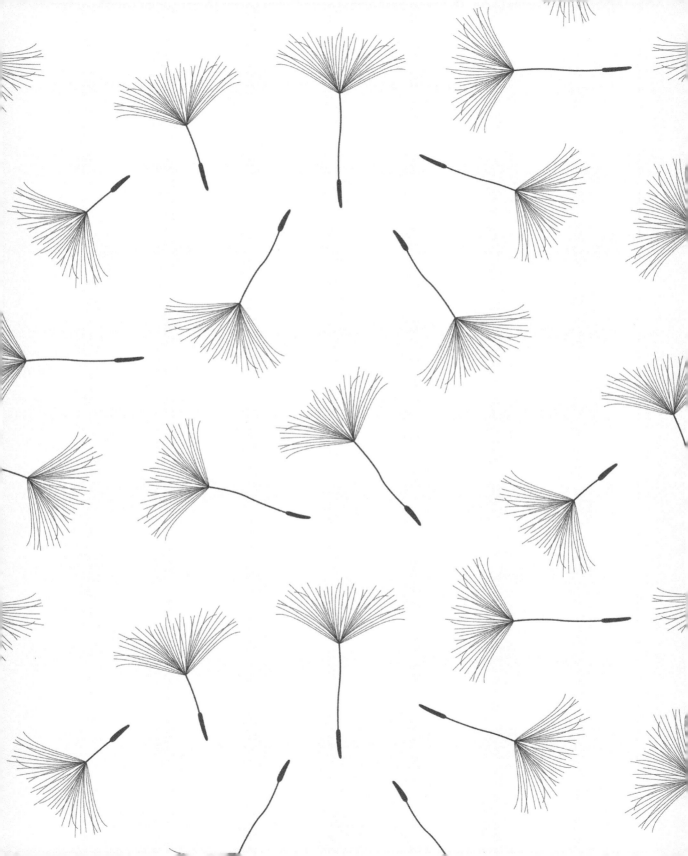

Chapter Five
Tracking Cervical Mucus

When we consider all available FAM techniques, monitoring cervi-cal mucus is the primary method that best helps chart ovulation and time intercourse. Though the idea is off-putting to some women, it is a relatively simple technique. You may already be doing it if you've noticed changes in your vaginal discharge throughout the month. In this chapter, we'll discuss the relevance of cervical mucus—what it does, what it can tell us, and how to monitor its evolution through the cycle.

Let's start with what it does. Many women think of their cervix only when the time comes for their Pap test (or never). However, the cervix is incredibly important when it comes to fertility and pregnancy. Latin for *neck*, the cervix is the narrow cylindrical passage between the vagina and uterus. Though the average cervix is only two to three centimeters in length, the internal surface is lined by hundreds of glands producing mucus that changes substantially throughout the course of an ovulatory cycle. During infertile times, or on hormonal contraception, the mucus is thick, white, acidic, and relatively clumpy. These properties make it an effective barrier against sperm or bacteria trying to enter the uterus. This barrier is critically important in pregnancy, as the cervix develops a protective mucus plug to ward off infection.

As the ovarian follicle grows, it releases estrogen, and the consistency of the cervical mucus becomes more watery, stretchy, alkaline, and clear. This enhances sperm survival on the journey to fertilization. Along the way, the cervical canal is lined with small folds in the tissue that allow for a prolonged release of sperm. With these mechanisms, sperm is able to survive inside of the female reproductive tract for three to five days.

Why You're Charting Cervical Mucus

Cervical mucus plays a vital role in signaling impending ovulation and in assisting sperm to reach the ultimate site of fertilization, the Fallopian tube. The main advantage of cervical mucus monitoring is that the quality of mucus clearly signals when ovulation is about to occur—unlike other FAM methods, which reveal when ovulation has passed. It is an incredibly useful tool for cycle tracking.

Its value is particularly high for women whose cycles are not always the same length. As discussed in chapter 1, it is typically the first half, or the follicular phase, of the menstrual cycle that varies from woman to woman, or from month to month. Each new cycle presents an unknown time frame from period to ovulation. Calendar or temperature methods can only offer an estimate of the fertile window based on averages of prior cycles, but cervical mucus monitoring can identify the days leading up to ovulation. In other words, whereas other methods might correctly include your most fertile days, especially if you have consistent cycles, cervical mucus monitoring is the primary sign of events in the cycle as it happens.

Some women may grow concerned if they do not experience clear changes to their cervical mucus or if they notice changes over time. There are several factors that can influence the quality of cervical mucus, but you can also rest assured that women do frequently conceive without ideal cervical mucus. I would certainly recommend speaking with your physician if you have concerns or need help monitoring your cycles in the absence of clear cervical changes, but don't start to worry unnecessarily; there may very well be nothing wrong.

CERVICAL POSITIONING

As a supplement to tracking cervical mucus, a minority of women also track their cervical position. When I think back to my first year as a resident physician in obstetrics and gynecology, and consider how many gynecologic exams it took before I, my classmates, or any of the newly minted OB/GYN interns I subsequently supervised during my training, could reliably examine a cervix, I typically hesitate in recommending monitoring cervical position. It can be quite tricky! There is also a natural variation to vaginal length, so for some women, feeling their cervix may be particularly difficult. That said, some women do find it helpful, so if you want to try it, here's how.

Start by washing your hands and making sure your nails are trimmed short. To avoid advancing vaginal bacteria into the cervix, I would avoid this method if you are actively dealing with a yeast infection, bacterial vaginosis, or any other vaginal irritation or infection. The best positions for checking your cervix would be sitting on the toilet, with one leg on a bathtub or chair, or while squatting. Then, insert your index or middle finger into the vagina until you feel the firmer texture of the cervix, somewhat similar to the tip of your nose. During your non-fertile days, the cervix will be relatively lower, firmer, and with a closed dimple for its opening. As you approach your ovulation, the cervix will move up higher, soften, and slightly open.

Keep in mind a few caveats: one, these differences are relative, so it will take a while to discern the difference. Two, unlike cervical dilation when you're in labor, the cervix barely opens. It is a subtle change! Three, if you have had a vaginal delivery before (or if your cervix was dilated in the process of a miscarriage, uterine surgery, or early labor, even if you ultimately had a Cesarean section), the cervical opening at baseline will be slightly larger and shaped more like a narrow slit, rather than the round dimple of a cervix prior to childbirth. When you remove your finger after checking, you may also find that you've obtained a good mucus sample to evaluate.

Remember, checking cervical positioning is an optional adjunct to tracking your mucus, but if you're searching for one more sign to help clarify your ovulatory status, it might be a good option for you!

Checking Your Cervical Mucus

How does one check cervical mucus? There are a few ways, depending on your com-fort level and the clarity of your body's signals. Let's start with the least invasive option: observation. As you approach ovulation, the water content of your cervical mucus increases, and you may notice that you simply feel wet, as if you're sitting in a little puddle. You may also observe staining in your underwear. Early nonovulatory cervical mucus will clump, appear yellowish, or form linear streaks in your underwear. Ovulatory discharge forms a clear, round, thin stain, spreading symmetrically. For some women, especially after tracking their pattern for a few months, these signals can be a sufficient tip-off that ovulation is imminent.

However, the true method of cervical mucus monitoring does involve actually checking your mucus. With this technique, be sure to wash your hands first, and keep your nails trimmed as well. Check whenever you feel comfortable. Begin by sitting on the toilet or resting one leg on a raised surface. Use toilet paper or tissue to spread your labia, and wipe front to back to collect any discharge that has settled. You can then examine the mucus from the tissue.

Alternatively, you can actually insert your index or middle finger into your vagina to try and reach closer to your cervix and sweep out any discharge present in the vagina. No matter how you collect the sample, once you have it, visually inspect the discharge by rolling it between your thumb and finger for texture, and finally separate your fingers to see if the discharge is stretchy or breaks apart easily. You can classify the discharge into one of four categories:

Not Ovulating (Dry/Sticky)

Once your period bleeding is finished and you can more easily assess your cervical discharge, you might find it to be sticky or rubbery in texture, relatively less abundant, and dry feeling overall. It will be opaque, white, or yellow in color. Keep in mind that if you have a short cycle or long duration of bleeding, your cervical mucus changes could overlap with your period, so you might start your monitoring at one of the next phases of mucus progression. Some women actually ovulate while they are still menstruating, so definitely seek evaluation if you cannot identify the shifts in your cycle.

Ovulation May Be Coming (Creamy)

As the ovarian follicle begins growing and estrogen levels begin to rise, the mucus becomes creamier, almost like a hand lotion. The texture is thinner than the dry, sticky mucus from the prior phase. The color will remain white-yellow but may start to look slightly less opaque.

Ovulation Is Close (Wet/Watery)

As follicular growth continues, the creamy mucus transitions into a more watery discharge. The fluid is increasingly wet and thin, and the color continues to lighten.

Ovulation (Wet and Stretchy/Egg-White Consistency)

As you enter the periovulatory window, the discharge will be at its most wet, thin, clear, and stretchy stage, most similar to raw egg whites. You might notice this discharge stretching for inches, either between your fingers or, if you're on the toilet, from your vagina down to the water. This mucus may slip out when you sit down to use the

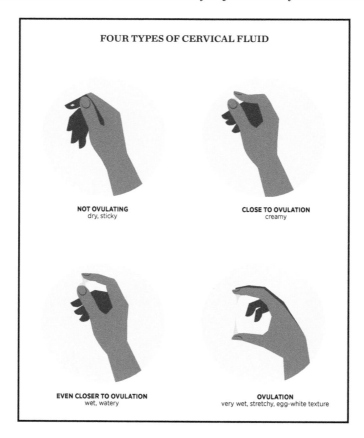

FOUR TYPES OF CERVICAL FLUID

NOT OVULATING
dry, sticky

CLOSE TO OVULATION
creamy

EVEN CLOSER TO OVULATION
wet, watery

OVULATION
very wet, stretchy, egg-white texture

toilet, but it will not dissolve into the water; rather, you may see it sinking down toward the bottom of the bowl. After ovulation, the secretion of progesterone will quickly cause mucus to dry up and return to the dry, sticky, nonovulatory phase.

Tips for Checking Mucus

If you are having difficulty obtaining a sample, try checking in the morning. Cervical discharge builds overnight so there may be more when you wake up. However, if you have intercourse at night the discharge may be related to ejaculate and/or arousal fluid. Use the restroom immediately after intercourse (lying in bed after sex does not increase your chances of pregnancy!) to reduce your risk of urinary tract infection and clear the discharge for a better read in the morning. You can also try checking after a bowel movement—sometimes this process helps move cervical discharge lower in the vagina—or try doing Kegel exercises prior to checking. This systematic tightening and relaxing of your pelvic floor muscles also helps move mucus and is an important technique for preventing urinary incontinence after pregnancy.

If you find yourself checking multiple times daily for days or weeks at a time without any visible progression in your discharge, it may be time to add in alternate methods of fertility awareness, seek professional guidance, and check for the presence of other factors that can influence your cervical mucus. Also remember that, though the goal of tracking mucus is identifying your fertile window and perhaps gaining insight into your cycle, many women conceive without ever being able to pick up cervical discharge progression. If you're having trouble, don't lose hope—get help instead.

What Else Affects Cervical Mucus?

As with other fertility awareness signs, cervical mucus monitoring is not completely foolproof. Other factors can impact the quality of cervical discharge as well as your ability to monitor changes. Any time you have concerns about the reliability of your technique, note the measurement as being possibly inaccurate. That way you will remember which observations you might need to exclude if they end up being outliers on your chart. Some of these factors may also be a sign that medical care is warranted, so keep an eye on them.

ANTIHISTAMINES
Antihistamines serve the purpose of drying up congested nasal and sinus passages during respiratory infections or allergic reactions. They are also associated with less abundant cervical discharge. Though one-time use is unlikely to have a significant impact, if you typically use antihistamines frequently and are concerned about the impact on your fertility, talk it over with an expert.

CLOMID

Clomiphene citrate (brand name Clomid) is a frequently used oral fertility medication. As a selective estrogen receptor modulator, it has both proestrogen and antiestrogen impacts throughout the body. In some women, it has marked antiestrogenic effects on the cervix or uterus. As a result, some women notice less cervical discharge and/or lighter period bleeding after taking clomiphene. Speak with your physician if you are noticing these side effects.

PCOS

The impact of polycystic ovary syndrome (PCOS) is covered more than once throughout this book, as it is the most common cause of absent or irregular ovulation. Relating to cervical discharge, women with PCOS may either never notice progression or, quite frequently, will notice a fluctuating pattern where the mucus appears to be moving toward ovulatory but never quite makes it, and just becomes dry again. Another observed pattern is where the discharge may even seem ovulatory and then dry up, but then become watery and abundant again within the next few weeks or before a period arrives. Because progesterone after ovulation would keep the mucus thick and dry for two weeks until a pregnancy is established or the next period comes, these fluctuating patterns all suggest ovulatory dysfunction and can be commonly observed in PCOS.

AROUSAL FLUID

As previously described, checking cervical discharge after intercourse is inadvisable due to the presence of arousal fluid and ejaculate. But the arousal fluid alone can throw off your observations, so checking for ovulatory status once aroused but prior to intercourse would be difficult as well.

VAGINAL AND CERVICAL DISCHARGE

There are many infectious or inflammatory situations that can cause increased production of vaginal or cervical discharge, including sexually transmitted infections (STI). If you've had unprotected intercourse with a possibly nonmonogamous partner, STI testing is important to make sure you're not at risk for any potential effects of uncured infections, including tubal-factor infertility. If the tubes do become dilated and damaged, they can sometimes collect fluid that spills out as watery vaginal discharge. It is also fairly common to have disruptions in the normal bacterial balance in the vagina, leading to yeast infections or a condition called bacterial vaginosis. Reactions to condoms, douches (which are disruptive to your vaginal microbiome and should be avoided), or menstrual hygiene products could also cause discharge. Finally, precancerous and cancerous changes in the cervix can also increase your discharge, so make sure you are up-to-date on your screening Pap test.

CREIGHTON VERSUS BILLINGS VERSUS MARQUETTE METHODS

Since the original discovery of the cervical mucus pattern, many methods have sprung up to codify it into a named technique. The Billings Ovulation Method (BOM) was the first such method. This technique involves recording a daily, subjective description of how dry or wet you feel and applying either a colored stamp or symbol to track your observations. You keep an eye out for the change from a dry to a wet sensation, which indicates a possibly fertile day. Once you have gotten the hang of tracking, you can apply the "four simple rules," which include avoiding intercourse while menstruating, alternating intercourse on infertile days (so that every other day readings are free of arousal fluid or ejaculate), and then, once a change is noted, waiting for observation of your peak fertility (your wettest, most slippery sensation). This method gives instructions for those trying to either achieve or avoid pregnancy, and tutors are available through the World Organisation of Ovulation Method Billings (WOOMB). Though WOOMB is not an inherently religious organization, this FAM method is approved of by the Catholic Church.

The Creighton Model is an even more complex system of observing and charting "fertile biomarkers," taught by trained instructors following a set curriculum. The method, developed for heterosexual couples at the Saint Paul VI Institute for the Study of Human Reproduction, is based in Catholic teachings. The Creighton Model is one component of what the institute refers to as NaPro (natural procreative) Technology, the ability to analyze your body's fertility markers, not only to assist with contraception or pregnancy but also to identify risks for possible gynecologic issues such as PCOS, endometriosis, and more.

Finally, the Marquette Method, developed at the (Catholic, Jesuit) Marquette University and approved of by the Catholic Church, uses a more technological approach to fertility monitoring. Practitioners of this method monitor their fertility via cervical mucus and basal body temperature, but the key distinction is that they also use a specific fertility monitor to track urinary estrogen and LH levels (urinary testing is discussed in more detail in chapter 8, page 121). The monitor identifies days of low, high, and peak fertility based on how high the hormones have risen. There are also courses available to assist couples in learning this method.

These three methods share the goal of strengthening the marital relationship through the joint investment of both partners in natural family planning. They offer varied degrees of assistance in educating women and couples, and interpreting fertility charts. For those who may share a moral or faith-based approach to FAM and are in a heterosexual marriage where both partners are invested in actively participating, or for those who simply want a more structured way to learn and practice FAM, these options can provide an incredibly rich and supportive community.

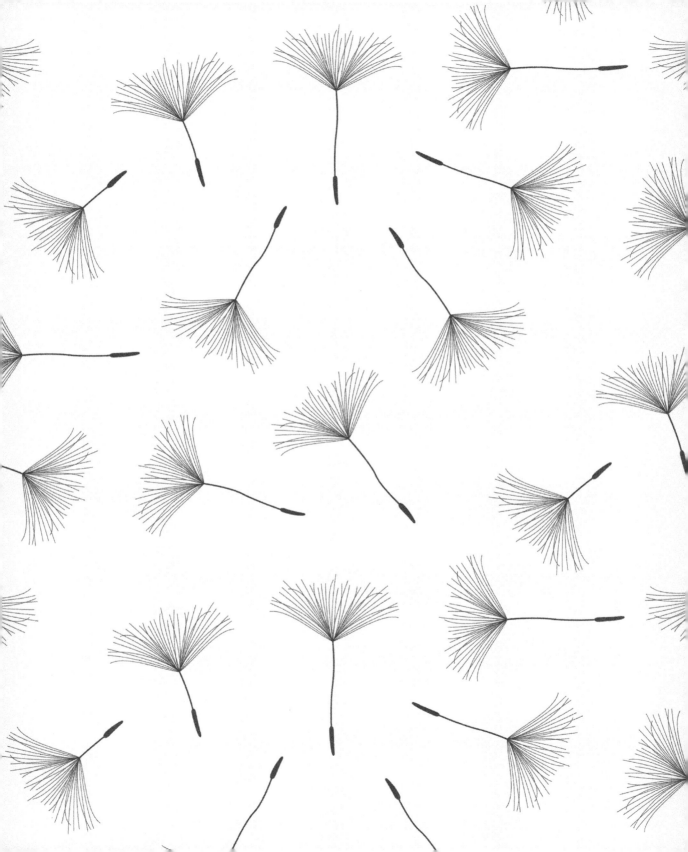

Chapter Six
Basal Body Temperature

In this chapter, we will take a detailed look at the basal body temperature (BBT) method of ovulation tracking. BBT tracking is one of the core FAM techniques and is the most effective method of FAM when combined with cervical mucus monitoring. For many women, it is an empowering method that delivers insight into their menstrual patterns and cycles. For this reason, even some women undergoing infertility treatment continue to monitor their temperatures. However, there are also a number of misconceptions and misunderstandings about BBT. For some women, temperature monitoring may also feel onerous or confusing.

This chapter will review the significance of BBT and how it relates to ovulation. It will discuss how to take BBT (it is slightly more complicated than you might think), what other factors can impact your basal temperature, and what your BBT tracking can and cannot tell you. It will focus on how to ensure you're tracking correctly and which patterns might indicate the need for further evaluation. For those who choose to monitor their temperatures, the exciting news is that in some cases BBT can even provide an early hint that a pregnancy is starting.

Why You're Charting BBT

Basal body temperature is a simple concept. It is your body's lowest resting temperature, reached after a night of restful sleep. Basal temperature is a more precise measurement than the way temperature is usually taken. It requires a specific thermometer that measures hundredths of a degree (two decimal points). The majority of women will experience a post-ovulation rise in their basal body temperature. Further, the absence of a temperature shift is highly likely to indicate an ovulatory or ovarian issue that needs further evaluation.

Aside from its proven effectiveness, there are many other reasons tracking BBT has become so popular. Once properly explained, it is a relatively simple technique that women can manage themselves with minimal technology. The data generated provides the basis for fertility charting and can be easily compared across cycles. Since it deals with an objective number, BBT tracking is less intimidating to some women than the more subjective assessments of cervical mucus or other fertility signs.

Finally, for some women, temperature tracking is part of creating a FAM lifestyle. As the first act of each day, it helps put you in the mindset of listening to your body and looking out for other signs of your reproductive and general health. This mindset of using the temperature-tracking ritual as a meditative moment to set an intention for a mindful, healthy, bodily aware day can be an empowering way to view BBT tracking. Indeed, many women share an appreciation for the closeness they feel to their inner reproductive lives through the monitoring of their temperature.

As a caveat, though, it would be remiss not to note that women can also find themselves incredibly frustrated with BBT, particularly those with irregular cycles, confusing temperature shifts, or infertility. This perspective is also completely understandable—it is difficult to start every day actively thinking about your fertility struggles. I hope that after reading this book, women will be able to identify whether they fall into one of these categories and feel empowered and motivated to seek help rather than feeling frustrated in isolation. Being told that a fertility specialist will help them monitor their ovulation—and thus they can stop checking their temperatures if they prefer—can be a big relief. No matter how you feel about BBT tracking, the goal of this book is to help you understand the available FAM options, choose the ones that are right for you, and recognize any signals your techniques are uncovering. Let's dive in.

What Does My Temperature Mean?

Now that we have discussed the importance of BBT in general terms, let's discuss specifically what your temperature can actually tell you. As covered in chapter 1, progesterone is an ovarian hormone produced by the corpus luteum after ovulation. The presence of progesterone raises our basal temperature so that the average basal temperature before ovulation is 97 to 97.5 degrees Fahrenheit, and 97.6 to 98.6 degrees Fahrenheit after ovulation. Though this rise is subtle—only 0.5 to 1 degree—and not a change you would expect to notice on your own, through temperature tracking you can observe these changes and note your pattern and ovulatory status over time. In a cycle not resulting in pregnancy, progesterone levels will drop, initiating the next period. As a result, temperatures will also drop down to the follicular baseline, often a day or two before the bleeding begins.

Thus far, it may seem quite simple. The tricky part, however, is that even within your follicular and luteal phases, there is daily variation. What you are actually looking for is a sustained rise of the average temperature that will last for the duration of the luteal phase. When you are first starting to chart, it will likely be at least three days before you might feel confident that your average has really shifted. Charts will be covered in much more detail shortly, but let's look at a brief example here. If you saw a temperature of 97 degrees Fahrenheit on cycle day 10, and 97.9 degrees Fahrenheit on cycle day 11, a rise of almost a full degree, you might think you've seen your temperature shift. However, in looking at the entire cycle, it might turn out that the average of cycle days 1 to 10 was 97.5 degrees, and that day 12's temperature dropped right back down to this number. So, no ovulation yet; day 11 was just a normal daily variation.

What you are really doing is monitoring your temperatures over the course of your entire cycle without homing in on any one daily value. You can also increase your confidence in interpreting temperatures by observing cervical mucus changes or other ovulatory signs and symptoms. After tracking this information for a few cycles, you might become quite familiar with your pattern and easily recognize your temperature shift right when it happens. This combined symptothermal method is the most efficient because, as discussed earlier, the cervical mucus can signal impending ovulation, whereas the temperature shift confirms ovulation has already happened. This is quite important, since by the time your temperature goes up, the fertile window has already closed. Thus, the primary value of BBT tracking lies in the initial confirmation that you do ovulate, especially if you have recently discontinued hormonal contraception or are unsure of your cycles, and in providing ongoing confirmation and clarification of your ovulatory pattern.

Some women will observe a slight temperature dip on the day of ovulation. Though this is relatively uncommon, if you observe this pattern after a few cycles, you're in luck—it is a bonus to get a prospective ovulation signal from BBT tracking. Temperature tracking can also offer some hints as to a developing pregnancy. Some women will note another temperature bump a week after ovulation, at the time of implantation. Though it will still be too early to detect pregnancy by blood or urine testing, such a pattern could hint at a positive test to come. However, even without this sign, temperatures that stay at the higher luteal levels longer than typical, without the drop that precedes the next period, are yet another sign of pregnancy. If you notice this, it may be time for a pregnancy test.

Taking Your BBT

In following chapters, we will work through some FAM charts and the intricacies of BBT interpretation. However, the monitoring must be done in a very specific manner in order to be accurate. Without reliable accuracy in your temperature measurements, your charting will not only be unhelpful, it might actually give you false information. So, let's discuss the most important details on how to take your basal temperature.

The first step is choosing a thermometer. As mentioned, the thermometer must have gradations to the 0.01 degree and generally will be labeled specifically as a basal temperature thermometer. A general-purpose thermometer you might already own to check for fevers does not have this precision. Basal temperature thermometers can be digital or glass, and either option is acceptable. Digital options may have memory recall or other advanced features you might prefer, though they typically cost more than a glass thermometer.

The other key factor is how the temperatures are taken—orally, vaginally, or rectally. It is easiest to start off taking oral temperatures, and most women can get reliable monitoring this way. If, after following the key steps described here, you find that your chart is difficult to interpret or your temperatures do not line up with your cervical mucus or other FAM signs, then it might be worth a trial in your next cycle using either a vaginal or rectal approach. For many women, a vaginal temperature may be easier or less intimidating to take, but go with whichever feels most comfortable to you. Just make sure that you take your temperature the same way for the entire cycle, as vaginal and rectal temperatures will typically be higher than oral measurements. A consistent technique is essential.

You probably think you know how to take your temperature, but let's talk about it a bit. Digital thermometers are fairly straightforward: Put the thermometer under your tongue, close your mouth to prevent air circulation, and start the measurement. Keep the thermometer depressed under your tongue until it beeps. For vaginal or rectal temperatures, just ensure that the tip is fully inside your body, the majority of the thermometer stays outside, and be sure to clean your thermometer after each use. For glass thermometers, check to make sure you have shaken down the prior reading the night before and give the thermometer five minutes to take its measurement. Ideally you can note your temperature right after you take it, but if not, you can always record it later. Whether you use a digital thermometer that flashes the last reading when turned back on, or a glass one that you haven't yet shaken down, you should be able to access your last reading later in the day.

Having discussed the what and how, let's discuss the when. The basal temperature is lowest right upon waking, and that is when the temperature must be taken—first thing in the morning. You would be surprised at what brief activities can impact your readings, so make sure that checking your temperature is absolutely the first thing you do. Getting up to use the bathroom, cuddling with your partner, shaking down a glass thermometer with an old reading—all of these actions can alter your measurements. It may take some getting used to, but once you get in the habit, it can be easy to remember. Just take your temperature once and you are done for the day.

Changes and Challenges

Since reliable measurements are the number one necessity in BBT tracking, you'll need to be aware of external factors that can impact your basal temperature. Some women are very regular cyclers despite these factors, wheras others are not and can find their cycle shortened or lengthened depending on the circumstances. When you are starting out with BBT charting, in addition to recording your temperature, you should also jot down the presence of any of these factors. Eventually, with more data it will become clear what does and doesn't impact you. Keep in mind that, although we often talk about a FAM lifestyle, it is not expected or necessary to abstain from all of these activities. It is simply impossible to eliminate all stress or illness from your life, and many people travel with some regularity. The key is knowing which environmental influences could cause a reading to be inaccurate, and then learning how your body responds to those influences.

Illness or fever. Perhaps the most self-explanatory factor, illnesses can impact your temperature. Certainly a fever will make your charting unreliable, but as the body's immune system works overtime to fight off infection or other stresses to the body, the basal temperature can be higher or lower than usual. If you have had a recent infection or even a flare-up of a chronic illness, keep an eye out for any associated changes to your cycle.

Stress. Severe forms of physical or emotional stress can result in cycle alterations: earlier or later ovulation, reduced progesterone production, and even complete cessation of ovulation. When it comes to the stresses of daily life, there is significant woman-to-woman variation in the susceptibility of your cycle. Some women can recall cycle changes during stressful times in school or after a personal loss or challenge. These are hints at how our bodies respond to stress.

Night-shift work. Fluctuations in the basal temperature are driven by the circadian rhythm, which in turn depends upon the typical wake-sleep cycle. Working night shifts or having alternating day-night shifts disrupts this rhythm and may throw off your ovulation pattern and your ability to catch temperature changes, and possibly even increase the risk of miscarriage.

Interrupted sleep cycles or oversleeping. Similarly, your basal temperature being lowest in the morning depends upon at least three hours of sleep preceding the measurement. For women who wake frequently, or who may get up in the early morning hours to use the restroom, temperatures may be unreliable. On the other hand, oversleeping can also cause one to miss their lowest temperature and result in inaccurate readings.

Alcohol. Alcohol consumption from the prior night can also raise your basal temperature, impacting your readings. As with the other factors, there is no universal threshold beyond which you'll definitely be affected, so continue to track when you drink and how much so you can flag potentially problematic readings. Keep in mind that some data suggest that alcohol use, particularly with increasing frequency or binge-drinking, prolongs time to conception, so cutting down or abstaining from alcohol intake in the preconception phase is advisable.

Hot or cold rooms. The ambient temperature in the room or the use of heated blankets can also alter your temperature and therefore impact your readings, particularly if these habits change from day to day.

Travel and time zone differences. Time zone changes can result in a desynchronization between your circadian rhythm and your travel schedule. This and other altered habits or sleep environments while traveling can potentially contribute to inaccurate temperature readings.

Medications. Some medications can impact your basal temperature as well. This is certainly true for antipyretics and anti-inflammatory drugs, such as Tylenol, and nonsteroidal anti-inflammatory drugs (NSAIDs) like ibuprofen or naproxen. Some evidence suggests other medications, especially neurologic or psychiatric drugs, may also impact your temperature. In general, before conceiving, it is advisable to speak with your prescribing physician about all medications you take, not only to find out if they might impact your cycle but also to ensure that they are safe to be taken in pregnancy.

Gynecologic Disorders and Your BBT

As discussed in depth in chapter 2, there are certain gynecologic disorders that can throw off your cycle in a variety of ways. The end result, however, is the same: these conditions can complicate charting and the interpretation of your temperatures. Let's take a look at some of the most common issues.

The most obvious problem arises in those situations where ovulation never occurs. For women who have polycystic ovary syndrome (PCOS), the most common cause of absent ovulation, the irregular bleeding pattern is typically the first hint of a problem. That said, I have taken care of many women with PCOS who reported regular cycles that were subsequently found to be anovulatory. As previously stated, this pattern will show up in a cycle that shows no rise in temperature. Alternatively, some women with PCOS do ovulate, but often sporadically, so the chart may show a very prolonged follicular phase with low temperatures—even months at a time—followed by a sudden ovulation and temperature rise.

For women trying to conceive, this pattern is incredibly frustrating because of its unpredictability and how long it might take to ovulate. Though I would recommend seeking help and exploring treatment options if this is your pattern, while tracking at home you may also want to start monitoring for other fertile signs because—remember!—your BBT chart will not alert you to an impending ovulation, and you don't want to miss your shot.

Alterations in other hormones, like your thyroid or prolactin hormones, can also disrupt your ovulatory pattern. These diagnoses sometimes manifest with associated symptoms: feeling constantly fatigued or cold, brittle hair or hair loss, or weight gain for low thyroid levels; or headaches, visual changes, or breast discharge for high prolactin levels. Again, if your charting demonstrates prolonged phases without ovulation, it is definitely important to ensure there are no medical explanations.

In cases where the ovulatory drive is suppressed due to high levels of exercise, stress, or restrictive eating, called hypothalamic amenorrhea, the big clue is that the period starts to become increasingly light and then stops altogether. In the absence of ovulation, the temperatures will stay low. Some women can be on the cusp of this phenomenon; a very active or stressful schedule can also lead to cycles where ovulation occurs but with reduced secretion of ovarian hormones. Blunted progesterone production could show up as a temperature that is slow to rise or is imperceptible by temperature tracking.

This slow or unclear rise in temperature could also be a result of diminished ovarian reserve, where we see lower follicle quantity and quality as a result of age or other diagnoses. In these cases, we see similarly lower ovarian hormone production, and can therefore see these abnormal patterns. Additionally, it is common with diminished reserve to see a shortening follicular phase, meaning that ovulation can occur increasingly earlier in the cycle. In some cases, women may see ovulation occurring before their period ends. This pattern is problematic and another reason to seek evaluation, because the uterine lining has not had sufficient time to develop by the time an embryo might be present for implantation.

Finally, endometriosis can also have an impact. Though ovarian endometriosis can cause diminished ovarian reserve, the most commonly mentioned side effect is elevated temperatures during the period. This pattern is caused by the prostaglandin activity and inflammation present during this time, which is also responsible for the painful period cramping characteristic of endometriosis. If you notice temperatures that either drop at the end of the luteal phase and then rise again during the bleeding, or that do not drop until the period ends, particularly if combined with other signs of endometriosis, further evaluation can help confirm the diagnosis or rule out any other symptoms of the diagnosis, such as blocked tubes or ovarian cysts.

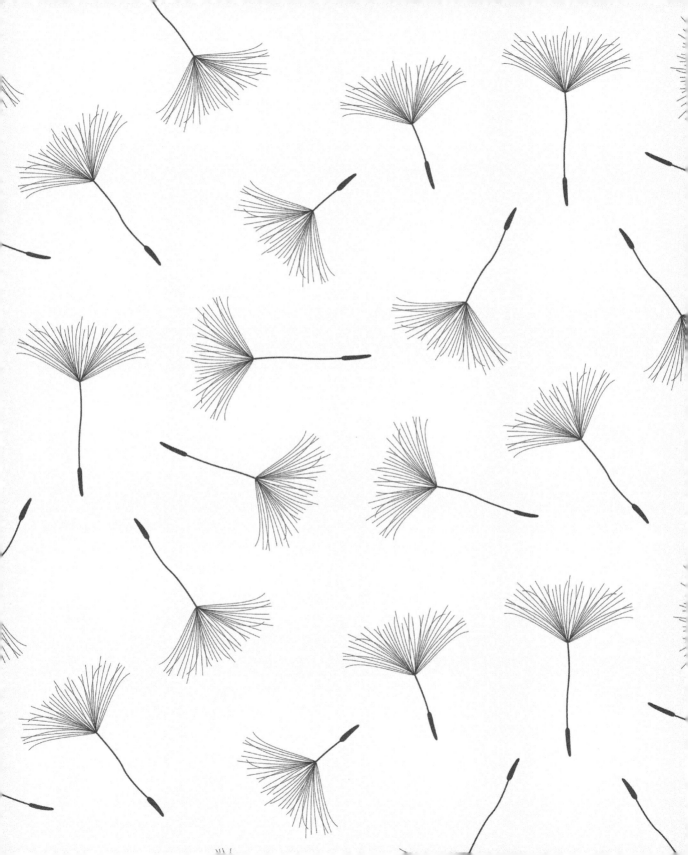

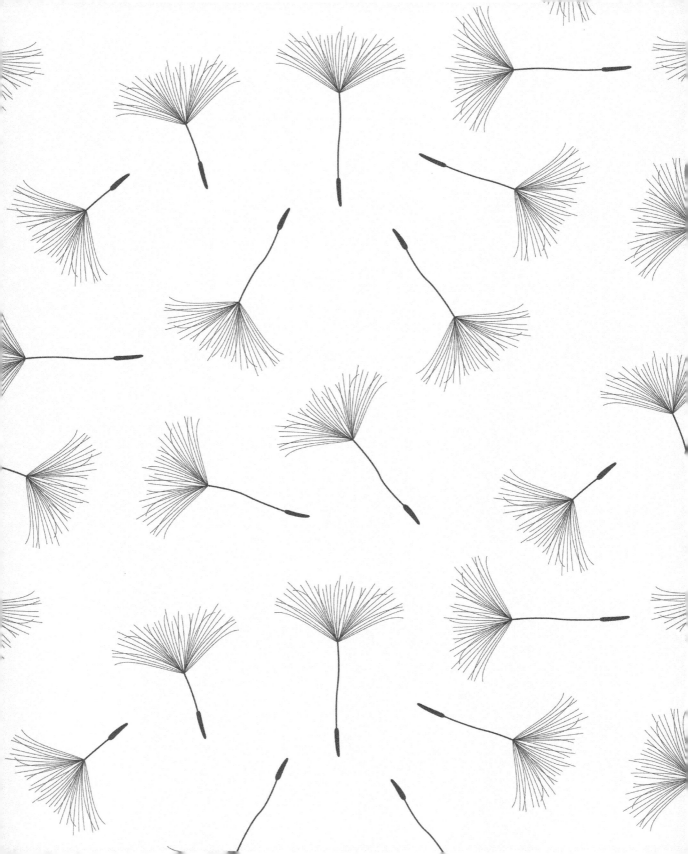

Chapter Seven
Charting and Tracking Your FAM

Now that you have all the information, let's put everything together to show how FAM charting may look for you. Tying together the data you can get from calendaring, tracking temperatures, and cervical mucus, this chapter will review some common chart patterns and some of the most typical abnormalities.

The goal of this chapter is to try to make the day-to-day process of FAM come to life and, most importantly, feel approachable and doable. For many women, once they get the hang of cycle tracking, monitoring these basic parameters becomes second nature. However, for some women, some or all of their signs may simply seem confusing or fail to follow a predictable pattern. Even if you are one of those cases, by reading this far you will be able to identify when the data you are charting is in conflict or difficult to interpret. Later in this chapter, we will discuss some additional physical signs you can utilize to help analyze your cycle. Chapter 8 covers the technological options you might also consider for additional insight.

If at any point you find yourself struggling with the FAM method, remember you always have additional options. You might decide to go deeper into charting and pursue FAM tutoring via one of the intensive methods mentioned in chapter 3, or to see a fertility specialist for assistance interpreting your cycle and to assess the need for treatment. Some women become frustrated and exhausted after spending months or years trying to understand their cycle or achieve a more "normal" cycle on their own. You don't have to wait until your breaking point.

Finally, remember that if you are transitioning off of hormonal contraception, it may take some time for your cycles to settle into a pattern that you can track. This recovery can vary based on your body and on the type of contraceptive used, as discussed in chapter 2. But after six months or more, it is entirely reasonable to enlist some help if you have questions about your cycle and tracking progress to date. The message throughout this book is simple: When it comes to FAM and cycle tracking, you never have to struggle alone.

Reading Your FAM Chart

Now we will dive into a variety of sample charts that help illustrate and tie together all the techniques and signs we have been discussing for the past few chapters. We will demonstrate a few different methods of tracking, and learn not only how they might confirm ovulatory status and help identify your fertile window, but also how your FAM chart can indicate the potential for relevant gynecologic diagnoses and suggest that it's time to visit with your gynecologist or a fertility specialist. There is a lot of information that can be gleaned from tracking these symptoms, so let's see how we can interpret these signs!

Sample Chart

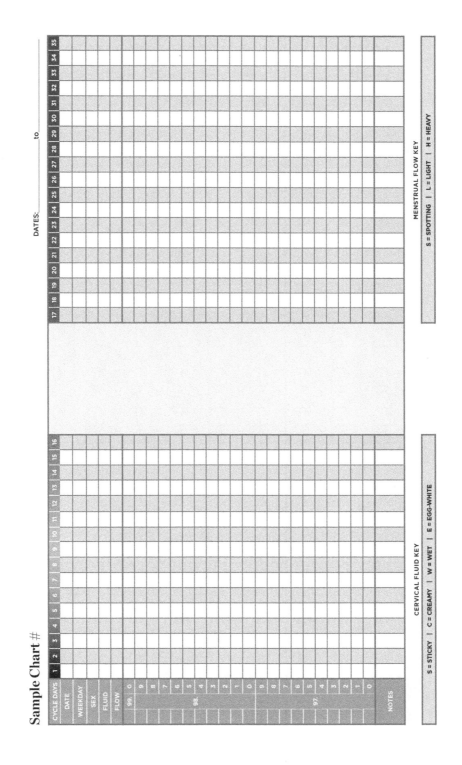

DATES: _____ to _____

CYCLE DAYS	1	2	3	4	5	6	7	8	9	10	11	12	13	14	15	16	17	18	19	20	21	22	23	24	25	26	27	28	29	30	31	32	33	34	35
DATE																																			
WEEKDAY																																			
SEX.																																			
FLUID																																			
FLOW																																			

NOTES

CERVICAL FLUID KEY

S = STICKY | C = CREAMY | W = WET | E = EGG-WHITE

MENSTRUAL FLOW KEY

S = SPOTTING | L = LIGHT | H = HEAVY

CHARTING AND TRACKING YOUR FAM   75

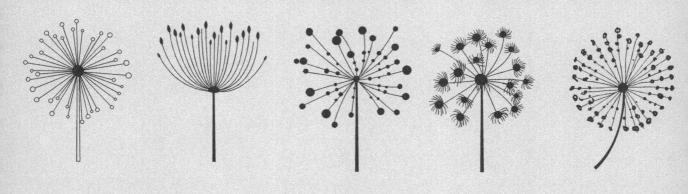

Understanding Fertility Awareness Methods

Sample Chart 1

This chart depicts the "textbook" 28-day menstrual cycle. The menstrual bleeding follows a normal pattern, with three heavier days followed by two lighter flow days and ending on day six with spotting. On day six, cervical mucus is still noted to be sticky. On days 10 to 12, the mucus transitions to creamy, watery, and then egg-white by days 13 and 14. By day 15, her basal body temperature has shifted upward, confirming ovulation on day 14. The luteal phase lasts a normal 14 days.

This chart is the most straightforward, without any conflicting signs or cycle abnormalities. Remember, only a small minority of women truly have a "clockwork" 28-day cycle. That said, many women might have regular cycles that are 27 or 29 days in length. In those cases, the changes in cervical mucus and temperature would correspond by shifting a day earlier or later, respectively. If you have a pattern where your cycle is fairly regular but varies within a day or two of your average cycle length, you can see how your ovulation day will also shift slightly, but tracking your cervical mucus will help alert you to the most fertile days for that particular cycle, with confirmation from a rising temperature.

Sample Chart #1

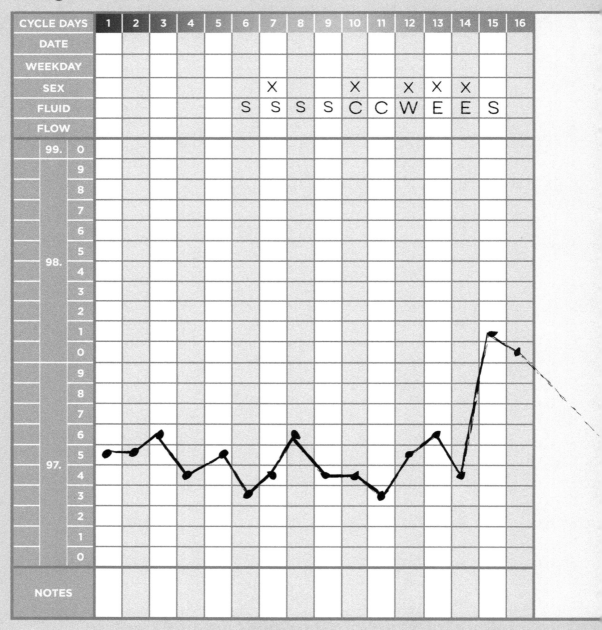

CYCLE DAYS		1	2	3	4	5	6	7	8	9	10	11	12	13	14	15	16
DATE																	
WEEKDAY																	
SEX								X		X		X	X	X			
FLUID							S	S	S	S	C	C	W	E	E	S	
FLOW																	

CERVICAL FLUID KEY

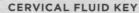

S = STICKY | C = CREAMY | W = WET | E = EGG-WHITE

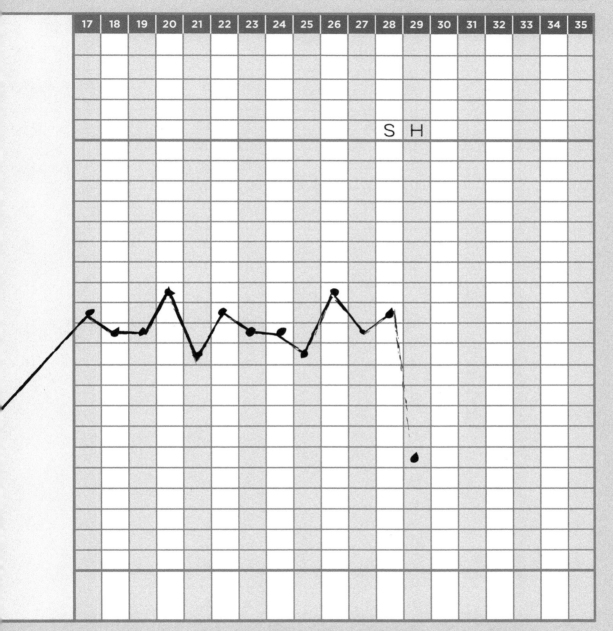

MENSTRUAL FLOW KEY

S = SPOTTING | L = LIGHT | H = HEAVY

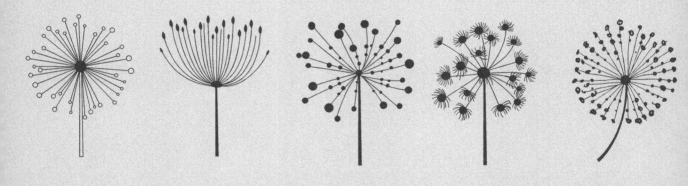

Understanding Fertility Awareness Methods

Sample Chart 2

This chart demonstrates a short follicular phase that results in a similarly short 24-day cycle. The menstrual bleeding follows a normal pattern with two days of heavier flow, one day of lighter flow, and one day of spotting. In this case, the choice was made to track dry versus wet vaginal sensations rather than cervical mucus characteristics. Also, unlike the other sample charts, this woman prefers to chart vaginal sensation and intercourse throughout the whole cycle, rather than just up to presumed ovulation with temperature rise. On day five, after the period has ended, she still feels dry, and this continues until days 9 and 10, which are characterized by vaginal wetness. Basal body temperature tracking shows a temperature rise on day 11, suggesting ovulation on day 10. The luteal phase is normal, lasting 14 days in length.

The pattern shown here is that of a normal, but relatively shorter, follicular phase. If a woman with this pattern was counseled to prioritize intercourse in the middle of her cycle (day 12) or on day 14 (which would be more appropriate for a 28-day cycle), she would be missing her ovulation. Therefore, we can see with this chart how understanding the different distributions of time in the follicular phase and the luteal phase, and recognizing the signs of impending ovulation, can be critical to timing intercourse appropriately.

It is also helpful to note that even though some women always have a shorter cycle, others see their cycles shift with age. As they approach their late 30s and early 40s, many women will find their cycle shorten by a few days. This shift occurs as the dominant follicle actually starts growing in the luteal phase of the preceding cycle. We see this frequently when women come in for an ultrasound early in their follicular phase and the lead follicle is already visible. As a result, ovulation occurs sooner. This slight shortening depicted here is not problematic as long as it is recognized. The Diminished Ovarian Reserve chart on page 105 shows a more extreme version of this trend.

Sample Chart #2

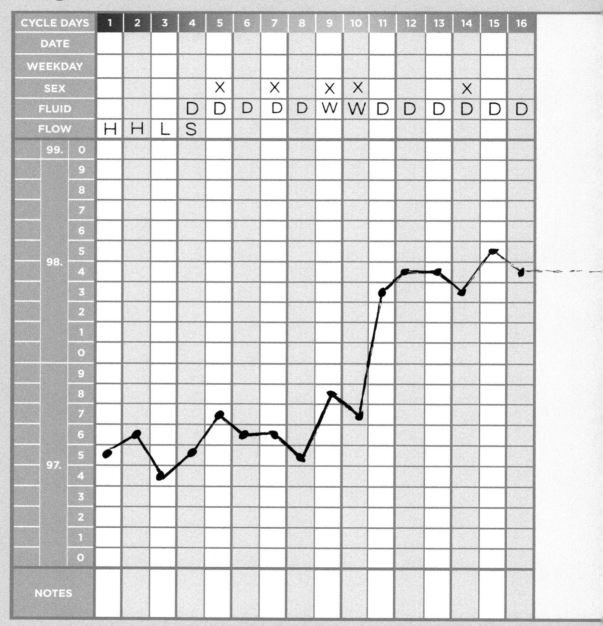

CYCLE DAYS	1	2	3	4	5	6	7	8	9	10	11	12	13	14	15	16
DATE																
WEEKDAY																
SEX					X		X		X	X				X		
FLUID				D	D	D	D	D	W	W	D	D	D	D	D	D
FLOW	H	H	L	S												

CERVICAL FLUID KEY

S = STICKY | C = CREAMY | W = WET | E = EGG-WHITE

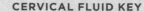

17	18	19	20	21	22	23	24	25	26	27	28	29	30	31	32	33	34	35
X				X														
D	D	D	D	D	D	D	D											
								L										

MENSTRUAL FLOW KEY

S = SPOTTING	L = LIGHT	H = HEAVY

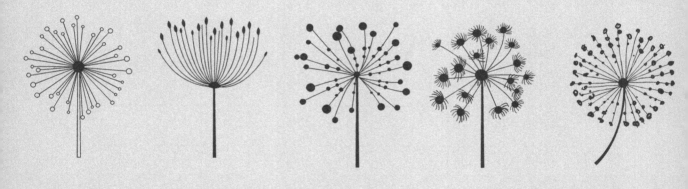

Sample Chart 3

This chart demonstrates the opposite pattern, that of the long follicular phase. In this particular chart, you can see a normal menstrual bleeding pattern, with three days of heavy flow, one day of lighter flow, and one day of spotting. The cervical mucus is sticky and remains that way until day 13, when it transitions into a creamy texture for days 14 to 16, watery on day 17 and egg-white on day 18. There is some slight spotting noted on day 18 as well. A temperature shift is noted by day 20, and a normal 13-day luteal phase follows. The overall cycle is therefore long, at 33 days.

The pattern shown here is also relatively common. Remember, the normal menstrual cycle can last anywhere from 24 to 38 days, so although ovulation appears to have occurred late on day 18 or 19, this cycle is not abnormal. The cervical mucus and temperature signs all line up accordingly. In this chart, you can see that sometimes the ovulatory signs span a day or two in length. This woman may have noted abundant egg-white cervical mucus on day 18 and felt sure that ovulation was impending. However, when the temperature had not yet risen on day 19, she realized that there could still be one more fertile day even though the mucus seemed somewhat diminished. After the eventual temperature rise on day 20, a normal luteal phase is noted as well. One more interesting note on this chart: Ovulatory spotting is another normal phenomenon some women notice. It is worth seeking assistance if this spotting turns into outright bleeding, but light spotting is not a cause for concern.

Sample Chart #3

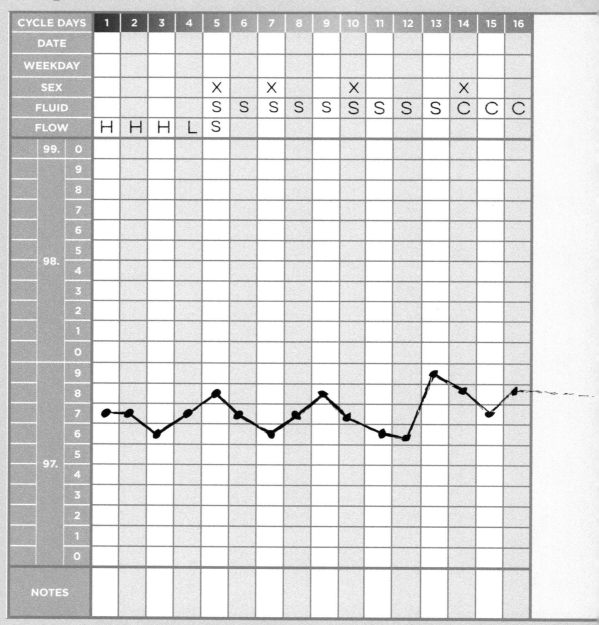

CYCLE DAYS		1	2	3	4	5	6	7	8	9	10	11	12	13	14	15	16
DATE																	
WEEKDAY																	
SEX						X		X			X				X		
FLUID						S	S	S	S	S	S	S	S	S	C	C	C
FLOW		H	H	H	L	S											

CERVICAL FLUID KEY

S = STICKY | C = CREAMY | W = WET | E = EGG-WHITE

17	18	19	20	21	22	23	24	25	26	27	28	29	30	31	32	33	34	35
X	X	X																
W	E	C	S													S	H	
	S																	

MENSTRUAL FLOW KEY

S = SPOTTING | L = LIGHT | H = HEAVY

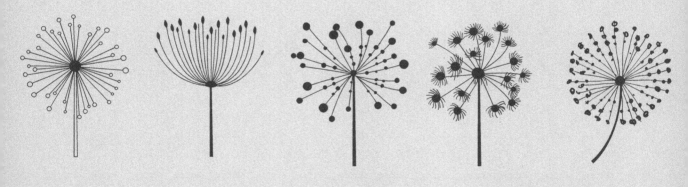

Understanding Fertility Awareness Methods

Sample Chart 4

This chart demonstrates another short cycle, in this case due to a short luteal phase. In this particular chart, we see a normal menstrual bleeding pattern, with two days of heavy flow, one day of lighter flow, and one day of spotting. The cervical mucus is sticky and remains that way until day nine, when it transitions into a creamy texture for day 10, watery on days 11 and 12 and egg-white on day 13. A temperature shift is noted on day 14. However, nine days later, some spotting is noted. By the next day, the temperature seems to already be dropping, and by 11 days after the presumed ovulation, the next period has started. Overall, the cycle is on the shorter side, at 24 days.

This chart shows what appears to be a normal follicular phase lasting 13 days. From the day of ovulation, we would expect either a positive pregnancy test or the next period about 13 to 14 days later. In this case, however, spotting started around nine days later. Luteal spotting can sometimes represent implantation spotting, which is discussed in the next example, but in this case it was followed by a dropping temperature the next day and full menstrual flow two days later, signaling that the spotting was simply a precursor to the next period. In total, the luteal phase only lasted about 10 days. It is important to recognize that, though this chart and chart 2 both show 24-day cycles, the timing of ovulation and the underlying hormonal patterns and key cycle events dictating the fertile window and cycle length are very different.

There can be many reasons for a short luteal phase. If the pattern is a one-time aberration, it is often due to stress or illness at the time. However, if the pattern is persistent, it is a sign that the follicle is not producing enough progesterone to hold off the next period for the full length of a normal menstrual cycle. In this case, various treatment options should be considered. A fertility specialist can help review these options with you, including supplements or various pharmaceutical approaches that can help support a robust luteal phase.

Sample Chart #4

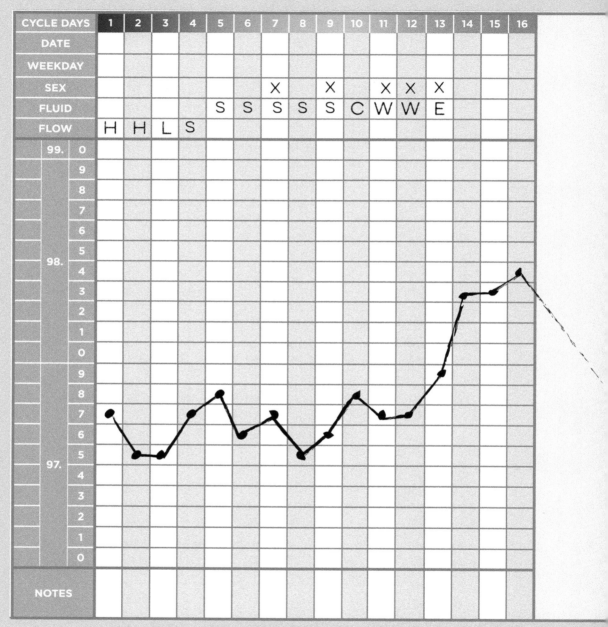

CYCLE DAYS	1	2	3	4	5	6	7	8	9	10	11	12	13	14	15	16
DATE																
WEEKDAY																
SEX							X		X		X	X	X			
FLUID						S	S	S	S	C	W	W	E			
FLOW	H	H	L	S												

CERVICAL FLUID KEY

S = STICKY | C = CREAMY | W = WET | E = EGG-WHITE

DATES:_____to_____

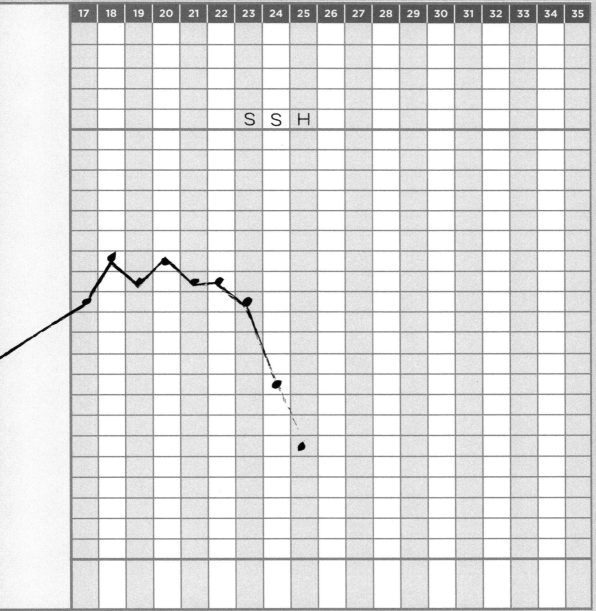

| 17 | 18 | 19 | 20 | 21 | 22 | 23 | 24 | 25 | 26 | 27 | 28 | 29 | 30 | 31 | 32 | 33 | 34 | 35 |

S S H

MENSTRUAL FLOW KEY

S = SPOTTING | L = LIGHT | H = HEAVY

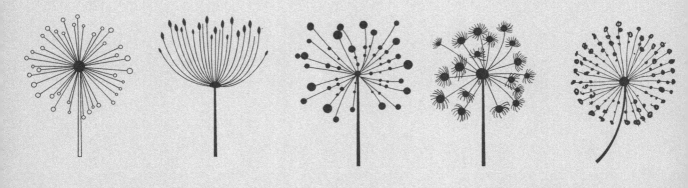

Understanding Fertility Awareness Methods

Sample Chart 5

Here is a chart that at first glimpse seems to start off resembling chart 4. It shows a normal menstrual bleeding pattern with two days of heavy flow, one day of lighter flow, and one day of spotting. The cervical mucus is sticky and remains that way until day 9, when it transitions into a creamy texture for day 10, watery on days 11 and 12 and egg-white on days 13 and 14. A temperature shift is noted on day 15. Again, nine days later, some spotting is noted. However, the spotting lasts only a day, and at the same time the woman's temperatures seem to shift even higher. By cycle day 28, without any further bleeding, a pregnancy test is taken, and is positive.

This is a classic pregnancy chart. Again, the follicular phase appears quite normal, and there is spotting that starts in the luteal phase. This timing can represent what is shown in chart 4, namely an abbreviated luteal phase and an impending period. However, women trying to conceive often hope that what they are observing is actually implantation bleeding. The concept is simple: As the embryo burrows into the uterine lining, it can disrupt some of the superficial blood vessels, leading to spotting or bleeding. Though some women will report this bleeding to be darker than their normal menstrual flow, observations of implantation bleeding are highly variable. Implantation bleeding may or may not occur, and it can vary in appearance or heaviness. Furthermore, implantation bleeding can take place at any point in the second half of the luteal phase (about 7 to 14 days after ovulation), and it is sometimes accompanied by cramping. Though it will typically be lighter and only last a few days at most, implantation bleeding can't be confidently confirmed until the pregnancy hormones can be detected.

Finally, some women experience a progesterone level that rises above their baseline luteal level with pregnancy. This hormonal bump can lead to the three-phase (triphasic) temperature pattern seen in this chart, where the temperatures rise with ovulation and then again halfway through the luteal phase, as seen here. Sometimes this progesterone bump can also lead to additional symptoms such as breast tenderness, but again, these symptoms are highly variable and often absent even in cycles where pregnancy is achieved.

Sample Chart #5

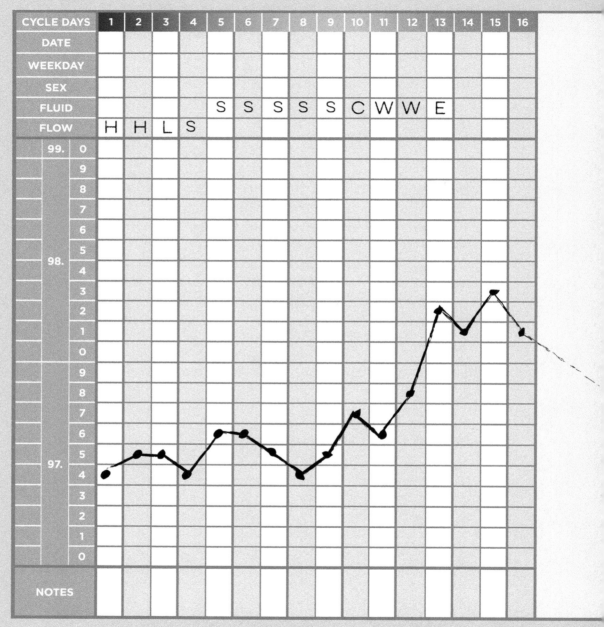

CYCLE DAYS	1	2	3	4	5	6	7	8	9	10	11	12	13	14	15	16
DATE																
WEEKDAY																
SEX																
FLUID						S	S	S	S	S	C	W	W	E		
FLOW	H	H	L	S												

CERVICAL FLUID KEY

S = STICKY | C = CREAMY | W = WET | E = EGG-WHITE

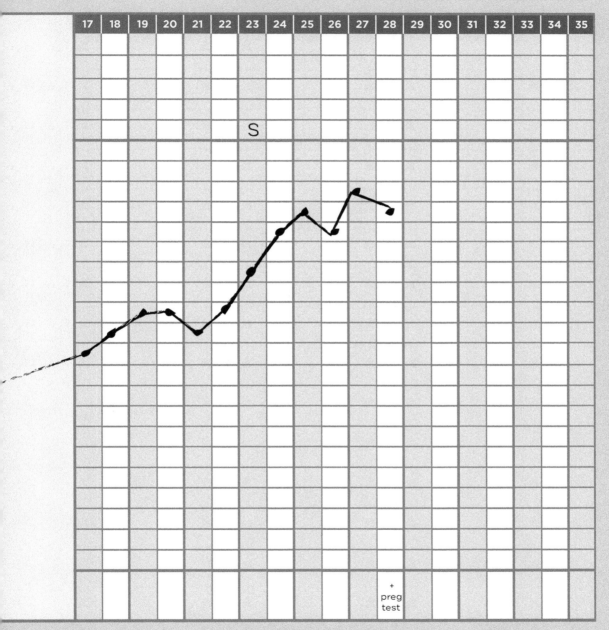

| 17 | 18 | 19 | 20 | 21 | 22 | 23 | 24 | 25 | 26 | 27 | 28 | 29 | 30 | 31 | 32 | 33 | 34 | 35 |

MENSTRUAL FLOW KEY

S = SPOTTING | L = LIGHT | H = HEAVY

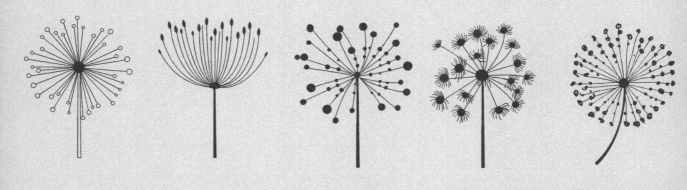

Understanding Fertility Awareness Methods

PCOS Chart

This chart is a typical pattern of an anovulatory cycle, where an egg is never released. Here, after a week of heavy bleeding, there are seemingly random fluctuations in cervical mucus and basal temperatures for 39 days before full-flow bleeding begins again. This pattern is most consistent with polycystic ovary syndrome (PCOS), where the brain secretes hormones to stimulate follicular growth, and some estrogen is produced by the abundant follicles, but the estrogen never rises to the ovulatory levels that can generate fertile signs, such as egg-white cervical mucus. As a result, the cervical mucus can sometimes seem like it's beginning to transition, but then may revert back to dry and sticky. In this pattern, due to the absence of ovulation, a temperature shift will not be observed. Eventually, the thickening uterine lining may trigger bleeding even despite the lack of ovulation, but a so-called anovulatory bleed will typically come outside of a 24- to 38-day window, be variable from cycle to cycle, and feature heavy prolonged bleeding. Some women with PCOS do ovulate, whether sporadically or with regularity, but this chart demonstrates the classic pattern with absent ovulation.

It is also worth revisiting the discussion in chapter 2 about possible causes of absent ovulation. For example, in women with hypothalamic amenorrhea, where the reproductive system shuts down due to stress, low body weight, excessive exercise, or restrictive eating, estrogen levels stay low throughout the cycle. In such a case it would be more likely to observe steady infertile signs without the fluctuations seen in this chart. Specifically, cervical mucus would likely stay dry and sticky throughout, without any temperature shift. These cases are also less likely to result in spontaneous bleeding, as the uterine lining typically stays quite thin. Regardless of what is causing the abnormalities, if your charting leads you to suspect an anovulatory pattern, it is worthwhile to seek evaluation, not only for fertility but to also address any associated risks depending on the diagnosis.

Sample Chart/PCOS

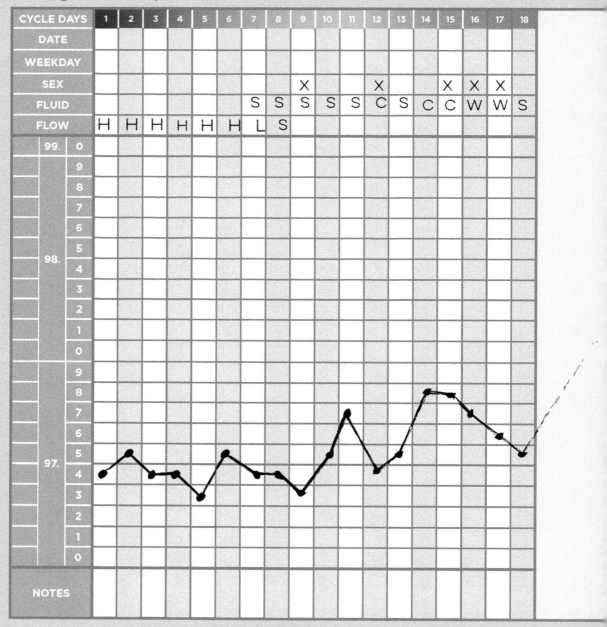

CYCLE DAYS		1	2	3	4	5	6	7	8	9	10	11	12	13	14	15	16	17	18
DATE																			
WEEKDAY																			
SEX										X			X			X	X	X	
FLUID								S	S	S	S	S	C	S	C	C	W	W	S
FLOW		H	H	H	H	H	H	L	S										

CERVICAL FLUID KEY

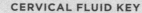

S = STICKY | C = CREAMY | W = WET | E = EGG-WHITE

DATES:_____to_____

19	20	21	22	23	24	25	26	27	28	29	30	31	32	33	34	35	36	37	38	39	40
				X		X				X			X					X			
S	C	S	S	C	C	W	C	S	S	W	S	S	C	C	S	S	S	S	S		
																					H

MENSTRUAL FLOW KEY

S = SPOTTING | L = LIGHT | H = HEAVY

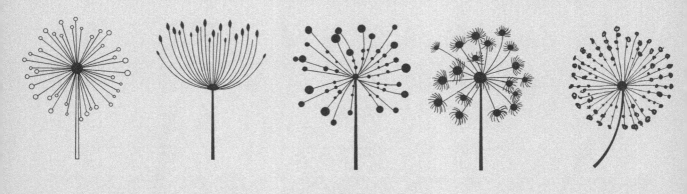

Understanding Fertility Awareness Methods

Endometriosis Chart

As we have discussed, when it comes to which FAM methods you use and which signs or symptoms you chart, there are many options. For women who experience pain, mood shifts, or other troubling symptoms throughout their cycles, charting these symptoms can be illustrative and help identify a pattern. This chart demonstrates what pain symptom charting can look like. The most classic symptom of endometriosis is painful periods, often so severely painful that the pain necessitates absent days from school or work. Another classic symptom is pain with intercourse, particularly with deep penetration, which puts pressure on tender areas of endometriosis inside the pelvis. Here we see that the pain and inflammation during the period likely contributes to a higher temperature during this time, dropping only after the period ends. Finally, two or more days of premenstrual spotting, as seen here on cycle days 28 to 30, is also highly associated with endometriosis.

Therefore, this chart, with severe cramping pain during the period, uncomfortable intercourse, and premenstrual spotting, is highly suggestive of endometriosis. Making these connections is important because studies have shown that diagnosis is often delayed, sometimes taking a decade or more before women are officially told they have endometriosis. Further, historically, exploratory surgery was part of the basic infertility workup, but once it became clear that this approach does not increase pregnancy rates, routine surgery was dropped. As a result, recognizing and communicating the signs in your cycle that may suggest endometriosis can help you get a diagnosis in a timely fashion.

Sample Chart/Endometriosis

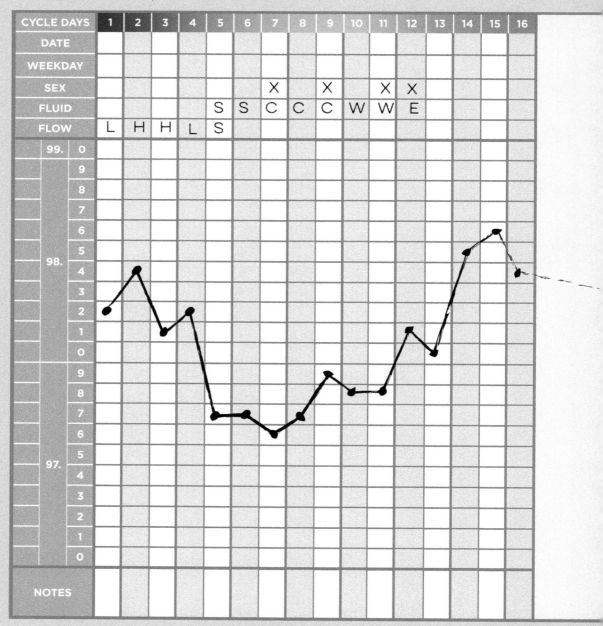

CYCLE DAYS		1	2	3	4	5	6	7	8	9	10	11	12	13	14	15	16
DATE																	
WEEKDAY																	
SEX								X		X		X	X				
FLUID						S	S	C	C	C	W	W	E				
FLOW		L	H	H	L	S											

CERVICAL FLUID KEY

S = STICKY | C = CREAMY | W = WET | E = EGG-WHITE

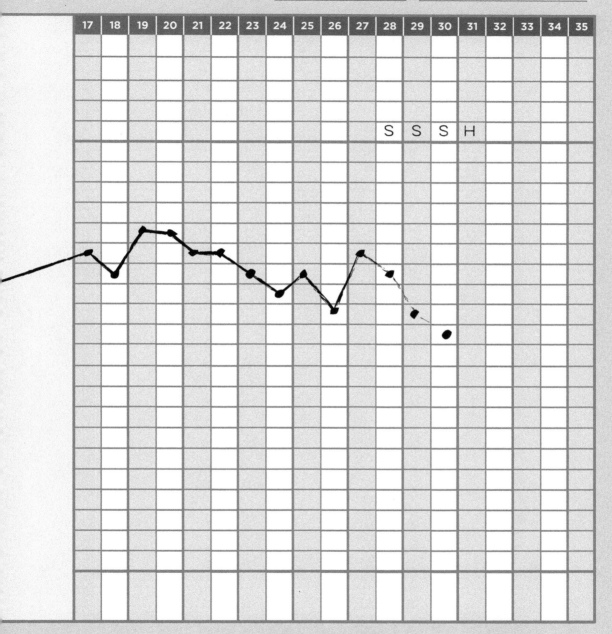

17	18	19	20	21	22	23	24	25	26	27	28	29	30	31	32	33	34	35
											S	S	S	H				

MENSTRUAL FLOW KEY

S = SPOTTING | L = LIGHT | H = HEAVY

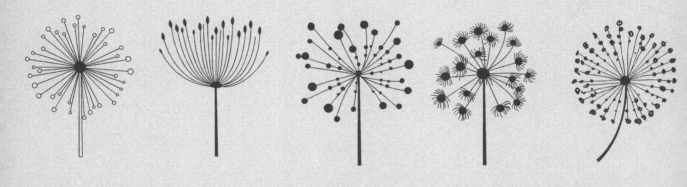

Understanding Fertility Awareness Methods

Diminished Ovarian Reserve Chart

This chart shows a pattern that suggests diminished ovarian reserve. This diagnosis refers to the quantity and quality of the follicle cohort. It is diagnosed when the number of follicles available to grow each month is lower than expected, with abnormal hormone levels suggesting reduced ovarian activity, or when there is a poor response to prior treatment. Age is the key risk factor, as ovarian reserve naturally declines over time.

This chart shows a few characteristics that suggest a diminished ovarian reserve diagnosis. As with chart 2, often a dominant follicle establishes itself early, even starting to grow during the preceding menstrual cycle, which results in ovulation also occurring quite early in the cycle. If this happens before the uterine lining has had sufficient time to grow, pregnancy is very difficult to achieve. If the dominant follicle itself is not of high quality, it may also be unable to generate sufficient amounts of estrogen and progesterone to produce the typical symptoms used with FAM. Indeed, this is what is shown here. The period is on the lighter side of normal, with three days of medium flow and then a day of spotting. Once the bleeding subsides, creamy cervical mucus is already noted. Without seeing a clear progression to egg-white, temperature shifts suggest ovulation occurs on day six or seven, though the luteal temperatures have just barely risen. The lack of ovulatory cervical mucus, along with low luteal progesterone levels, suggest poor follicle quality.

This pattern is one for which I would strongly recommend medical evaluation. Ovulating just a few days after menstruation has stopped and FAM signs that suggest both low estrogen and progesterone levels all point to a diagnosis of diminished ovarian reserve. At this point, diagnostic confirmation and consideration of treatment would be the best course of action.

Sample Chart/DOR

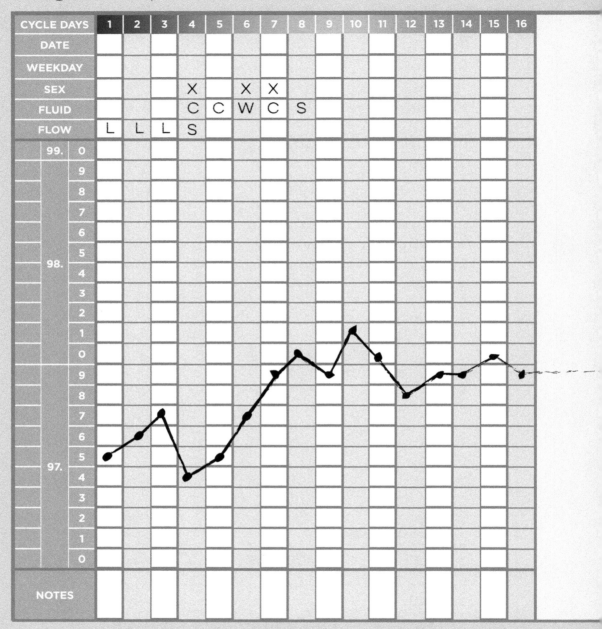

CYCLE DAYS		1	2	3	4	5	6	7	8	9	10	11	12	13	14	15	16
DATE																	
WEEKDAY																	
SEX					X		X	X									
FLUID					C	C	W	C	S								
FLOW		L	L	L	S												

CERVICAL FLUID KEY

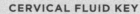

S = STICKY | C = CREAMY | W = WET | E = EGG-WHITE

17	18	19	20	21	22	23	24	25	26	27	28	29	30	31	32	33	34	35
			S	S	H													

MENSTRUAL FLOW KEY

S = SPOTTING | L = LIGHT | H = HEAVY

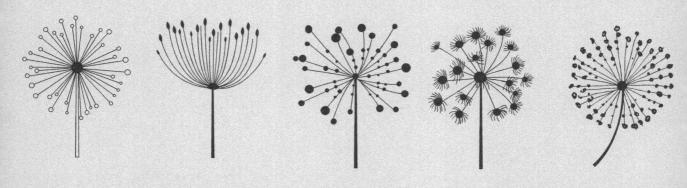

Understanding Fertility Awareness Methods

Miscarriage Chart

This chart demonstrates an early miscarriage. The cervical mucus and basal temperatures suggest ovulation on day 13. Not having seen any bleeding on the day she anticipated her next period to come, and seeing sustained elevated temperatures, this woman took a pregnancy test, which showed a faint positive. She repeated it for the next two days, and it seemed to be slowly darkening, or showing more positive. However, the following day she noted her temperature dropping. That evening, she experienced some cramping pain and by the next morning had heavy vaginal bleeding that appeared consistent with her period.

This pattern is referred to as a biochemical pregnancy. In this case an implantation begins and pregnancy hormone shows up in blood or urine testing, but the miscarriage occurs before the pregnancy is far enough along to be confirmed via ultrasound or microscopic evaluation of the miscarriage tissue. Because these biochemical losses typically occur early and, depending on how far they progress, may not generate pregnancy symptoms, they can easily be missed. In this case, the total cycle lasted 31 days, which, if not for FAM tracking, could have been misinterpreted as no pregnancy, just a slightly late period due to ovulation occurring a few days later than it actually did. Without knowing the date of ovulation, this woman would not have known exactly when to start testing for pregnancy and may have missed the miscarriage altogether. Though the guidelines for recurrent miscarriage focus on losses that occur slightly further into pregnancy, if you've experienced two or more biochemical pregnancies, you should still seek evaluation to rule out any diagnoses that could put you at risk for more miscarriages.

Sample Chart/Miscarriage

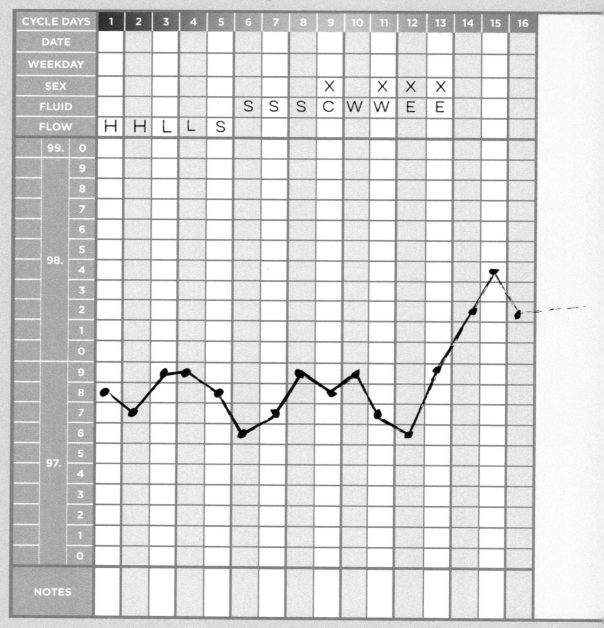

CYCLE DAYS		1	2	3	4	5	6	7	8	9	10	11	12	13	14	15	16
DATE																	
WEEKDAY																	
SEX										X		X	X	X			
FLUID							S	S	S	C	W	W	E	E			
FLOW		H	H	L	L	S											

CERVICAL FLUID KEY

S = STICKY | C = CREAMY | W = WET | E = EGG-WHITE

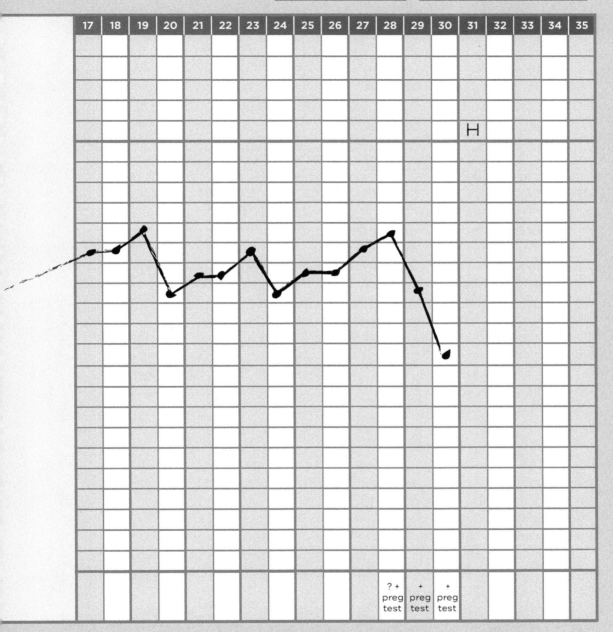

17	18	19	20	21	22	23	24	25	26	27	28	29	30	31	32	33	34	35

H

| | | | | | | | | | | | ? +
preg
test | +
preg
test | +
preg
test | | | | | |

MENSTRUAL FLOW KEY

S = SPOTTING | L = LIGHT | H = HEAVY

How to Read Conflicting Signs

When starting to use FAM, the concepts of monitoring often seem relatively straight-
forward. Sometimes, however, the data is confusing to interpret or seems in conflict.
In those instances, it is important to understand how to work through the signs you're
seeing. Of course, it's worth keeping in mind that the more types of FAM data you
incorporate, it is increasingly likely that one might not sync up with the rest at some
point. However, there are also more tiebreakers to help you sort out the reality of
what's going on.

Perhaps the most common thing I see is regular cycles but no ovulation. Though
data suggests that this happens in well below 10 percent of women with regular 24- to
38-day cycle lengths, it certainly occurs and is often a big surprise. In this scenario,
my patient will come in reporting cycles that seem to come quite regularly, and ini-
tially we may presume that this pattern signifies ovulation. If she has only been using
a calendaring method, we may discover the lack of ovulation incidentally through the
initial testing or treatment phases. Other times, a patient may come in because, despite
regular cycles, she has never been able to document changes in cervical mucus or basal
temperature. In that latter case of conflicting signs, there are a few key ways to confirm
ovulatory status.

One approach is to incorporate charting additional signs. There are many symptoms
associated with ovulation, but they tend to vary from woman to woman so it takes time
to recognize which ones you experience. These include increased libido, heightened
sense of smell, breast tenderness, and/or abdominal cramping. If you feel comfortable,
you might learn to check cervical position as discussed in chapter 5 (page 56). Finally,
premenstrual symptoms (again, quite variable from woman to woman) can at least
serve the purpose of suggesting ovulation did occur, even if they don't identify the
timing of the fertile window. Another approach, which is more common, would be to
add in some of the technological options discussed in chapter 8. These methods use
saliva or urine specimens to check for rising estrogen or LH levels consistent with ovulation. Finally, with the help of a physician, one could choose to monitor for follicular
growth via ultrasound, or check blood progesterone levels in the presumed luteal phase
for confirmation of ovulation. It's important to remember that calendar methods alone
are not the most precise, and cannot be trusted if they conflict with cervical mucus or
temperature tracking. However, there are many ways to troubleshoot that situation.

Another concern many women share is feeling that their cervical mucus never quite
reaches egg-white, and so they feel unsure of the exact timing of ovulation. In this
case, look to other signs to help confirm timing and presence of ovulation, especially
basal temperature. The limitation of temperature tracking is that it is a retroactive

confirmation, so if your cycle is a bit variable and you are pursuing cervical mucus monitoring to try and identify your most fertile days, not seeing a classic progression can be frustrating.

There are multiple options to resolve this. As demonstrated in the sample charts, some women prefer to simply note wet versus dry vaginal sensations. Others will check cervical position or, if they were checking mucus sitting at the vaginal opening, may attempt to collect mucus from deeper in the vagina for a better sample. You might also add ovulation predictor kits, discussed in chapter 8 (page 121). If, however, you notice additional signs similar to the diminished ovarian reserve chart, you may decide to seek evaluation and confirm that no additional treatment is recommended.

In short, if you are experiencing difficulty interpreting your charts, you can try at home to add in extra data points to pinpoint and confirm ovulation. If you find yourself struggling for six months or more, or sooner if you're highly suspicious of anovulation, it is definitely appropriate to seek some expert help so you can be sure about what is going on with your cycles.

When to Start a New Chart

Mistakes in charting are most common when you're first getting started and learning your body's unique signs. The most frequent errors include forgetting to chart regularly, taking your basal temperature incorrectly, confusing vaginal secretions or semen for cervical mucus, and misinterpreting mid-cycle spotting or bleeding for a new period. Let's discuss each of these briefly.

Charting insufficiently is likely the biggest issue if you're having difficulty interpreting your cycle. When you first get going, it is critical to note factors that might throw off your data, like stress, travel, illness, alcohol, and insufficient or interrupted sleep. It takes time to observe whether these variables influence your ovulation timing and/or basal temperatures. However, if you end up with a chart that has many questionable data points, it could be difficult to glean much from that particular cycle, and it might be worth starting again at a time when some of these extraneous factors can be minimized. You might also need a reminder to take your temperature first thing in the morning until you get in the habit, or to find some time in the day to chart.

If you're unsure at this point of your temperature tracking, go back to chapter 6 to review all the details of selecting a thermometer and testing. Taking your temperature even half an hour after waking up or after using the restroom can impact your results and contribute to a confusing chart. Similarly, if you're feeling confused about your cervical secretions, reread chapter 5 and decide if you need additional help in learning how to track your mucus progression. It is not uncommon for women to feel confused by the presence of semen, vaginal discharge, or lubrication fluid, but accurate mucus tracking requires you to be able to distinguish between these secretions.

Finally, if you do experience mid-cycle spotting or bleeding, it might be hard to tell when a new cycle has begun. Chances are, if it is solely spotting, it is not yet time for a new cycle. Day one of a new chart should only be assigned when full-flow menstrual bleeding is observed. Possible explanations for mid-cycle spotting are discussed throughout this book, including issues like endometrial polyps or the normal phenomena of ovulatory or implantation spotting.

Give yourself the grace and patience to find the process frustrating at first. If you're committed to using FAM, be sure you can at least regularly track your bleeding, temperatures, and cervical mucus, and then consider additional signs or technological assistance, as discussed in chapter 8. Again, read through the example charts for signs that it is time to get an expert opinion on your cycle.

Charting FAQs

Why aren't my days matching up with the sample chart?

The sample charts represent nine possible cycles out of infinite combinations of tracking data. Rather than trying to match up the days exactly, look for the pattern that most closely resembles your cycle to help you interpret what you're observing.

Why isn't my temperature rising?

If you've been using a basal thermometer correctly and you're not noticing a temperature rise, you may not be ovulating. Being anovulatory is even more likely if your cycle is irregular or falls outside of a 24- to 38-day length. There are many ways to confirm your ovulatory status, so consider seeking professional guidance.

Did I ovulate too close to my period?

By looking at the Diminished Ovarian Reserve Chart, you can see that if you ovulate within a few days of your period's completion, the uterine lining may not have enough time to generate sufficient thickness for implantation. If your chart suggests ovulation within two to three days or fewer of your period, you could consider ultrasound monitoring of your natural cycle to help confirm timing of your ovulation and assess the endometrial thickness at that time.

Help! I forgot to take my temperature before I got up. What should I do?

Forgetting to take your temperature is common, especially in the beginning. Go ahead and check your temperature, but note that it might be off. If it eventually looks like an outlier in interpreting your chart, you may choose to ignore it. Eventually, you'll learn what does and doesn't impact your temperature, and you'll become more confident about readings that weren't done under perfect circumstances.

I bled a little for a day and then I stopped. Do I start a new chart?

As previously discussed, mid-cycle spotting can occur for many reasons, and light bleeding is not usually cause for a new chart. Wait for your full-flow menstrual bleeding before starting a new chart. Keep in mind that if you are using an app for charting, you may not need to specifically assign a new cycle; rather, when you note full-flow bleeding, the app will automatically start a new cycle.

I am on hormonal contraception and hoping to be pregnant in the next year or so. When should I start charting my cycle?

Remember that while you're on hormonal contraception, you cannot chart your cycle. Depending on how strongly you feel about your pregnancy timeline, and whether you think you can properly use nonhormonal barrier methods for contraception, I often recommend stopping birth control three to six months prior to when you hope to get pregnant, and use that time to chart your cycles while using condoms or other barrier methods. In this way, once you feel ready to be pregnant, you'll already be armed with data on your cycle, and you will have given your ovaries time to start cycling again after the suppressive effects of birth control wear off. However, if you were on birth control for a specific reason—to control symptoms of endometriosis, for example—you may wish to discuss this with a physician first, as your symptoms may flare up once you stop birth control. Keep in mind that it is definitely possible to get pregnant right after coming off of birth control, so be sure to use protection until you're ready for pregnancy.

I just had a baby and am breastfeeding. Should I be charting my cycle?

Both the disrupted sleep and the hormonal suppression of ovulation while lactating are likely to throw off your FAM charting during the postpartum window. However, your first ovulation—commonly occurring around six months after delivery, though highly variable—will happen before the first true period, so be careful to use contraception to avoid another pregnancy so close to the previous one. Pregnancies less than 18 to 24 months from a prior delivery do run higher risks of complications, including preterm delivery, so if you're thinking of spacing your pregnancies closely, you may want to discuss the timing with your doctor. You can certainly resume charting at any point you like, but your symptoms will start to line up more clearly once you start ovulating, especially if you are getting some uninterrupted hours of sleep prior to your usual waking time.

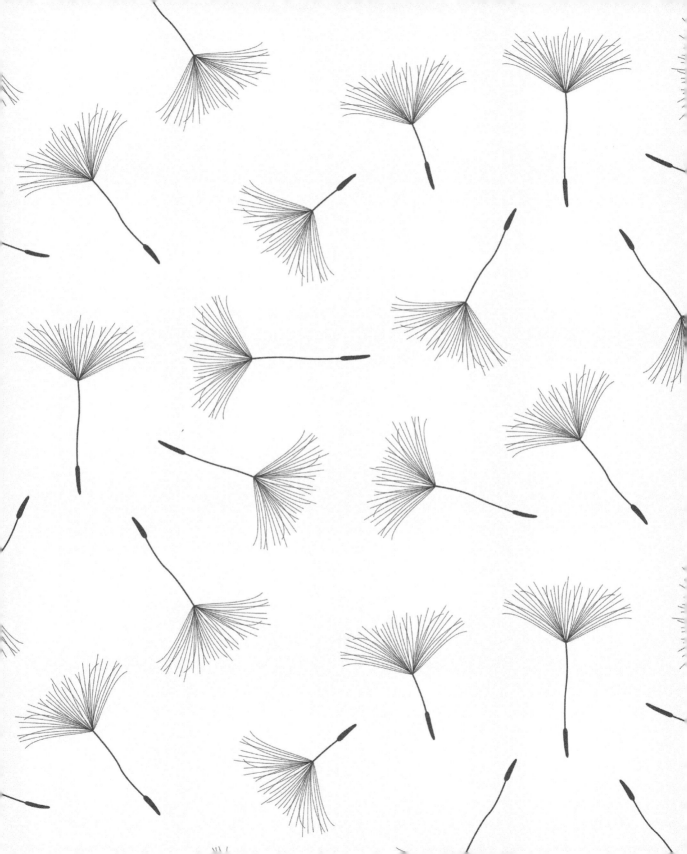

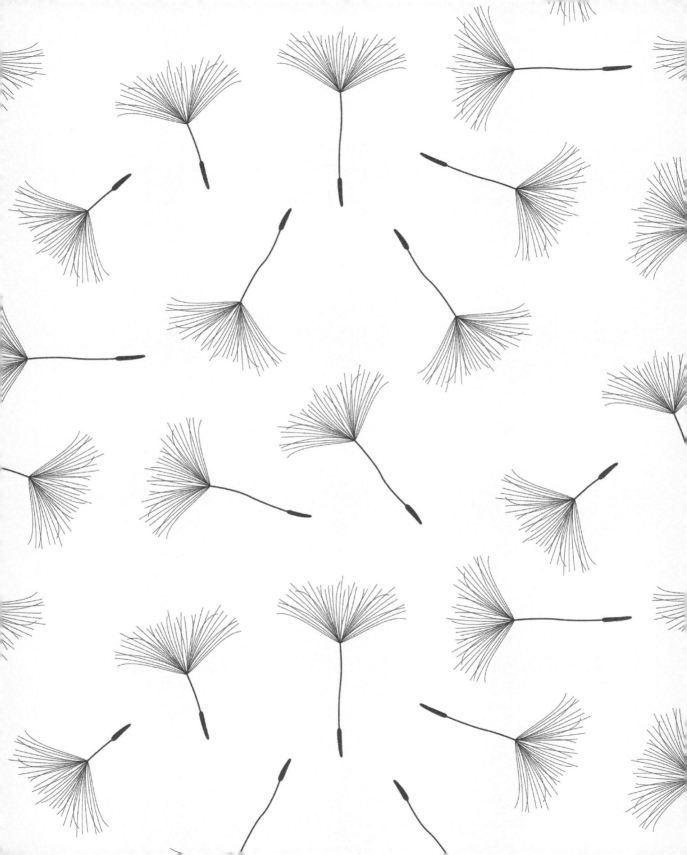

Chapter Eight
Tech Support for Your FAM

In the past few chapters, we have discussed the core FAM meth-ods in detail. Traditionally, women practicing FAM have charted on paper, using a template that includes all the signs they plan to monitor throughout their cycle. Of course, now there are many technological options that can help make the process of charting much simpler. These include websites and apps that assist with cycle tracking and fertile window prediction, smart thermometers and test kits for urinary and salivary hormones, and even wearable devices. Though these offerings are fraught with the same basic limitations as FAM itself, and are no guarantee of improved accuracy, they can provide additional insight into your cycle and/or assist with the process of charting.

Apps and Websites

The first offerings for technological FAM assistance were websites that offered a variety of charts, articles, online communities, and other resources. These include MyMonthlyCycles.com, FertilityFriend.com, and OvaGraph.com. The latter two options do have accompanying apps as well, and FertilityFriend.com is the official charting tool for Toni Weschler's book *Taking Charge of Your Fertility*.

There are also many smartphone apps on the market that can assist with FAM charting. These apps continually update their offerings, so here are some factors you might consider in selecting which app is best for you.

Tracking relevant to you. If you are planning to incorporate basal temperature or cervical mucus monitoring, make sure you choose an app that will take that data into account. Otherwise, the app's fertile window predictions will be less accurate than the information you're collecting. For example, the Clue, Natural Cycles, Kindara, and Period Tracker apps all allow for temperature tracking.

The look. FAM requires daily charting, so you will be using this app regularly. The aesthetic of the app may matter to you. Their interfaces range from clean and modern to pink and flowery. Select one that you feel excited using.

Scientific information. Some apps offer in-app scientific citations, associated blogs with additional helpful information, or even minicourses that can assist you on your FAM journey. Clue and Flo particularly excel in this area.

Privacy. Some apps have more discreet names or offer password protection to help keep your information private.

Syncing. Many apps offer the option for a partner to access your data, and the Glow app even has a companion male fertility tracker. Some apps can also be accessed via a smartwatch or fitness wearable.

Community. If you're interested in interacting with other women with similar family-building goals, an online community through the app may be valuable. Check out the types of forums they host to foster conversation.

Price. Almost all the good fertility apps have a free version, but many offer premium subscriptions or in-app purchases for additional services.

Here are some fertility apps that offer many of these features:

* Clue
* Cycle Tracking
* Cycles
* Dot

* Eve
* Flo
* Glow
* Kindara

* Natural Cycles
* Ovia
* Period Tracker by GP Apps

Hormone Testing

Hormone testing is another mechanism commonly used in conjunction with FAM approaches, particularly ovulation predictor kits (OPKs). As we have discussed in detail, one of the primary advantages of cervical mucus monitoring is that it can signal in advance your most fertile days for any given cycle. The progression of cervical mucus is dictated by the rising estrogen close to ovulation. However, the final surge of luteinizing hormone (LH) that directly causes ovulation does not create detectable symptoms. Therefore, the products discussed in the following section mainly use urine testing, but incorporate other data as well to help you catch your fertile window for that particular month in time to act.

As you read these offerings, you may begin to feel overwhelmed. What is now being called the "femtech" industry is actively exploding, and new products seem to come to market every few months. Some of the most advanced products can be expensive, so before investing in these gadgets, consider a few facts. First, as of yet, there is no scientific literature to prove that these devices offer a higher chance of pregnancy than traditional FAM techniques. Some of the newest ones may not even have published data on their efficacy. Second, if you have irregular cycles, missed ovulation, or other gynecologic issues, the limitations we have previously discussed will still apply. These tests are not foolproof and are not guaranteed to be accurate. So, if you utilize some of these options and are still not successful in conceiving, or are still confused about your cycle, definitely work with your physician to confirm your pattern. I have seen many patients come in with inaccurate data obtained from both OPKs and advanced fertility monitors—so use this technology if you find it interesting, stress-reducing, or informative, but don't feel pressured to add yet another thing to your FAM to-do list.

Ovulation Predictor Kits (OPKs)

Ovulation predictor kits (OPKs) assess urine samples to detect the sharply rising LH levels close to ovulation. The simplest and cheapest OPKs are strips that turn darker shades of blue as LH levels surge. The disadvantage of these strips is that sometimes reading them can be challenging. However, there is a whole spectrum of more advanced options. One option is the digital kit. These kits typically either read +/- or show smiley faces to highlight the two days of peak fertility. More advanced OPKs, such as the Clearblue Advanced Digital Ovulation Test, also test estrogen levels. Because estrogen rises in the days leading up to the LH surge, this type of OPK can distinguish between low fertility days and the approximately four days per month of high (rising estrogen) and peak (high estrogen, LH surging) fertility.

The offerings for OPKs have expanded greatly in recent years. In addition to the classic LH testing, or even the LH and estrogen kits, there are now additional options. Some kits (such as Pearl) offer test strips for follicle stimulating hormone (FSH), and others (such as Proov) offer confirmation of rising progesterone after ovulation. The yield of FSH testing is probably the lowest out of all of your cyclic hormones, but the progesterone testing could be a useful supplement to basal temperature tracking and another way to confirm that ovulation has occurred.

Fertility Monitors

Taking the technology one step further are the fertility monitors now available. The Clearblue Fertility Monitor, the official monitor used in the Marquette Method, has a touchscreen interface that helps you track your urine samples for LH and estrogen levels, storing data for up to six cycles at a time. Similarly, the newer Mira Fertility Analyzer records your LH surge and will also offer estrogen- and progesterone-level tracking. The data syncs to an analyzer and app to help provide you with analysis of your hormone results.

Other fertility monitors assess different data to help pinpoint your fertile window. The OvaCue Fertility Monitor has oral and vaginal sensors to detect cyclic changes in your electrolytes, or the minerals, such as sodium and potassium, that are normally present at varying levels in all bodily secretions. OvaCue analyzes this data to alert you to possible high- and peak-fertility days.

Smart Thermometers and Wearable Devices

Additionally, a number of wearable devices have been developed to allow for poten-tially simpler temperature tracking, without the need for a daily morning check. The Tempdrop is a wearable bracelet that reads your nighttime temperatures to help confirm ovulation and calculate your presumed fertile window as it learns your pattern over time. However, there are also a number of wearable devices that claim to detect your fertile window prospectively. The Ava is a sensor bracelet worn at night to monitor your temperature, pulse and heart rate variability, respiratory rate, and rate of perfusion (the passage of blood through your circulatory system), to identify five days of your monthly fertile window. The OvuSense and Priya Sensor are vaginal sensors, also worn overnight, that monitor continuous core body temperature to detect signs of ovulation.

Saliva Ferning

Finally, salivary testing, such as the Fertile-Focus kit, offers a small home micro-scope under which you can look for the classic "ferning" pattern that signals the rising estrogen of the periovulatory window. As the estrogen levels rise, it causes the saliva to form crystalline patterns that look similar to the leaves of a fern plant. Once ferning is identified, ovulation should occur within 24 to 72 hours.

The Many Ways We Make a Family

One of the great joys of being a fertility specialist is helping educate women about their reproductive health and empowering them on their fertility journey. That means offering insight into the data women and their partners have been collecting at home, and turning the data into an action plan for moving forward. It also means normalizing their experience. With 15 percent of couples facing infertility, societal trends showing steadily increasing maternal ages, and more LGBTQ and single-parent families, the need for some assistance along the way is very common. Yet, studies have shown that access to fertility care is highly uneven. Fertility specialists tend to be clustered in cities, and insurance coverage varies by state and employer. Many folks who are struggling to get pregnant put off seeking fertility care because they are afraid of what they might find out, or because they assume treatment will have a high price tag or isn't covered by insurance.

As you might have guessed from reading this book, the message is simple: Knowledge is power. The initial fertility consultation is typically relatively affordable, and you should be told ahead of time whether you have coverage for any recommended testing or treatment. Once you have the information, you can determine how to move forward. It can look so different from family to family. It can be as simple as Alexis's case. She was 36 years old, with irregular menstrual cycles. She had been trying to achieve a regular ovulatory pattern for three years with supplements and a healthy lifestyle, but her cycles remained persistently abnormal. She decided to move forward with a medicated cycle to help a follicle grow and ovulate, combined with timed intercourse, and conceived on the second try.

Sometimes, the fix is conceptually simple, even if it takes a lot of work to get there. June came in at 34 years old, wondering why she hadn't gotten pregnant after four years of unprotected intercourse. She was feeling saddened seeing so many of her girlfriends start and grow their families. She had been charting her cycle for more than two years, adding in more methods as the months went by. At the initial consult, her question was simple: "Can you tell me what's wrong with me?" The pressure women put on themselves to achieve their fertility and pregnancy goals can become very heavy, and June was definitely feeling weighed down. In the evaluation, it turned out that her FAM had been correct all along, but her husband had an incredibly low sperm count. She had assumed that she must have been doing something wrong, when that was absolutely not the case. They had to save for a few months and take out a loan to go through a cycle of in vitro fertilization (IVF), but they were successful on their first try, with multiple healthy embryos stored for future siblings when the time came.

In other cases, other elements can be incorporated into the plan. I have so many patients looking to get pregnant who have very low ovarian reserve, or are well into their 40s, and many of them turn to IVF with a donor egg. In this case, donated eggs are taken from a younger woman and fertilized with the male partner's sperm, and the resulting embryo is transferred into the female partner's uterus. Though I often remind my patients that deciding to move forward with a donor egg is an emotional transition, the science behind it is fascinating. I love to talk about epigenetics, the science of how genes are turned on or off. It turns out that all the choices you make during pregnancy have a huge impact on your baby's health, even if the child doesn't share your genes. It's an amazing way for couples to be able to experience the joys of pregnancy, delivery, and breastfeeding. Other cases might involve a sperm donor, or a gestational carrier, a woman who has typically had her own children already and will carry the pregnancy for the intended parents.

Finally, I have worked with couples over the years who have decided to move away from fertility treatment and pursue fostering or adoption. Many of my patients have encountered folks along the way who heard of their struggles and said something along the lines of, "Well, why don't you just adopt?" That callous attitude ignores the reality that these choices can also be emotionally challenging and costly. That said, they are amazing options for building a family as well. Others might decide that their family is fine as it is, especially if they already have a child. There is no universally right answer; each family-building journey is unique. Ultimately, prospective parents should consider what it is that they truly envision: Is it being pregnant, giving birth, raising a child together, or something else? There can be many ways to make these visions come true, and sometimes it helps interventions like donor eggs or sperm, or a gestational carrier, feel more acceptable. This question is also a reminder that, whether a child comes into our lives through a spontaneous conception at home, fertility treatments, or adoption, it is not our genetics that tie us together, but rather the heartfelt desire to create and be part of the family we are building. Ultimately, I try to help my patients remember that children conceived or adopted after a fertility struggle are truly fortunate to be so highly desired by their parents. That love is at the center of all the ways we make a family, and it is what makes being a part of these journeys so amazing, every single day.

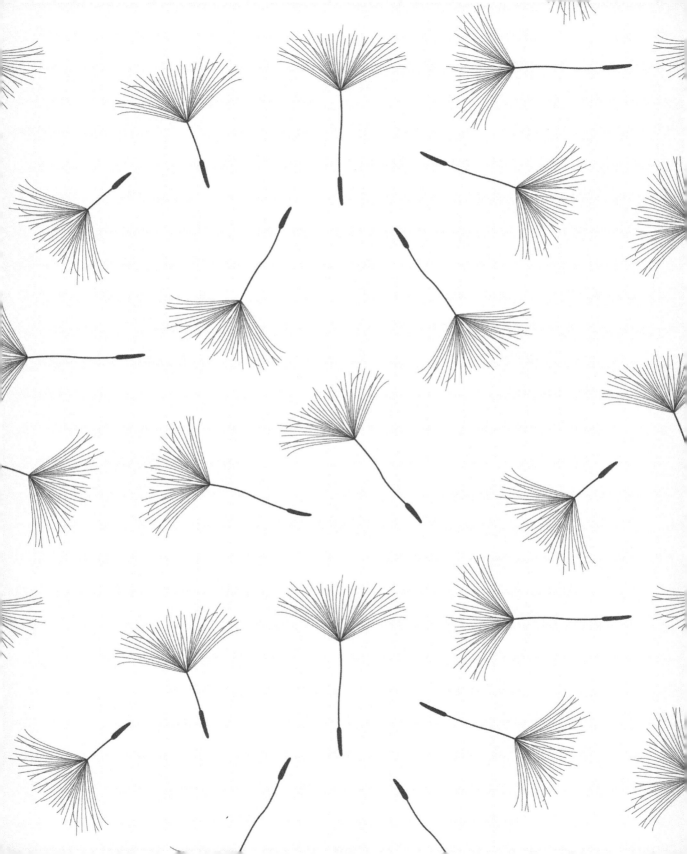

Blank FAM Charts

Sample Chart

CYCLE DAYS	1	2	3	4	5	6	7	8	9	10	11	12	13	14	15	16
DATE	04/06															
WEEKDAY	W															
SEX	—															
FLUID	P															
FLOW	M															
99. 0																
9																
8																
7																
6																
5																
98. 4																
3																
2																
1																
0																
9																
8																
7																
6																
5																
97. 4																
3																
2																
1																
0																
NOTES																

CERVICAL FLUID KEY

S = STICKY | C = CREAMY | W = WET | E = EGG-WHITE

	17	18	19	20	21	22	23	24	25	26	27	28	29	30	31	32	33	34	35

MENSTRUAL FLOW KEY

S = SPOTTING | L = LIGHT | H = HEAVY

Sample Chart

CYCLE DAYS	1	2	3	4	5	6	7	8	9	10	11	12	13	14	15	16
DATE																
WEEKDAY																
SEX																
FLUID																
FLOW																
99.	0																
	9																
	8																
	7																
	6																
	5																
98.	4																
	3																
	2																
	1																
	0																
	9																
	8																
	7																
	6																
	5																
97.	4																
	3																
	2																
	1																
	0																
NOTES																

CERVICAL FLUID KEY

S = STICKY | C = CREAMY | W = WET | E = EGG-WHITE

DATES:_____ to_____

17	18	19	20	21	22	23	24	25	26	27	28	29	30	31	32	33	34	35

MENSTRUAL FLOW KEY

S = SPOTTING | L = LIGHT | H = HEAVY

Sample Chart

CYCLE DAYS	1	2	3	4	5	6	7	8	9	10	11	12	13	14	15	16
DATE																
WEEKDAY																
SEX																
FLUID																
FLOW																
99.	0																
	9																
	8																
	7																
	6																
	5																
98.	4																
	3																
	2																
	1																
	0																
	9																
	8																
	7																
	6																
	5																
97.	4																
	3																
	2																
	1																
	0																
NOTES																

CERVICAL FLUID KEY

S = STICKY | C = CREAMY | W = WET | E = EGG-WHITE

DATES:_____to_____

17	18	19	20	21	22	23	24	25	26	27	28	29	30	31	32	33	34	35

MENSTRUAL FLOW KEY

S = SPOTTING | L = LIGHT | H = HEAVY

Sample Chart

CYCLE DAYS		1	2	3	4	5	6	7	8	9	10	11	12	13	14	15	16
DATE																	
WEEKDAY																	
SEX																	
FLUID																	
FLOW																	
99.	0																
	9																
	8																
	7																
	6																
	5																
98.	4																
	3																
	2																
	1																
	0																
	9																
	8																
	7																
	6																
	5																
97.	4																
	3																
	2																
	1																
	0																
NOTES																	

CERVICAL FLUID KEY

S = STICKY | C = CREAMY | W = WET | E = EGG-WHITE

DATES:_____ to_____

17	18	19	20	21	22	23	24	25	26	27	28	29	30	31	32	33	34	35

MENSTRUAL FLOW KEY

S = SPOTTING | L = LIGHT | H = HEAVY

Sample Chart

CYCLE DAYS	1	2	3	4	5	6	7	8	9	10	11	12	13	14	15	16
DATE																
WEEKDAY																
SEX																
FLUID																
FLOW																
99. 0																
9																
8																
7																
6																
5																
98. 4																
3																
2																
1																
0																
9																
8																
7																
6																
5																
97. 4																
3																
2																
1																
0																
NOTES																

CERVICAL FLUID KEY

S = STICKY | C = CREAMY | W = WET | E = EGG-WHITE

DATES:_____ to _____

	17	18	19	20	21	22	23	24	25	26	27	28	29	30	31	32	33	34	35

MENSTRUAL FLOW KEY

S = SPOTTING | L = LIGHT | H = HEAVY

Sample Chart

CYCLE DAYS		1	2	3	4	5	6	7	8	9	10	11	12	13	14	15	16
DATE																	
WEEKDAY																	
SEX																	
FLUID																	
FLOW																	
99.	0																
	9																
	8																
	7																
	6																
	5																
98.	4																
	3																
	2																
	1																
	0																
	9																
	8																
	7																
	6																
	5																
97.	4																
	3																
	2																
	1																
	0																
NOTES																	

CERVICAL FLUID KEY

S = STICKY | C = CREAMY | W = WET | E = EGG-WHITE

DATES:_____to_____

17	18	19	20	21	22	23	24	25	26	27	28	29	30	31	32	33	34	35

MENSTRUAL FLOW KEY

S = SPOTTING | L = LIGHT | H = HEAVY

Resources

There are an increasing number of books out there discussing fertility; the topics covered range from the nitty-gritty of menstrual cycles and using nonmedical approaches to troubleshooting your menstrual cycle. Although I cannot vouch for every detail in each of these books, overall they are well-regarded reads that can help provide more insight into your cycle and fertility. Some of these authors also have really robust social media accounts that offer useful information and inspiration.

Books

The Better Period Food Solution: Eat Your Way to a Lifetime of Healthier Cycles by Tracy Lockwood Beckerman

The Fifth Vital Sign: Master Your Cycles & Optimize Your Fertility by Lisa Hendrickson-Jack

Fix Your Period: Six Weeks to Banish Bloating, Conquer Cramps, Manage Moodiness, and Ignite Lasting Hormone Balance by Nicole Jardim

Healing Mind, Healthy Woman: Using the Mind-Body Connection to Manage Stress and Take Control of Your Life by Alice D. Domar and Henry Dreher

Healing PCOS: A 21-Day Plan for Reclaiming Your Health and Life with Polycystic Ovary Syndrome by Amy Medling

It Starts with the Egg: How the Science of Egg Quality Can Help You Get Pregnant Naturally, Prevent Miscarriage, and Improve Your Odds in IVF by Rebecca Fett

Making Babies: A Proven 3-Month Program for Maximum Fertility by Jill Blakeway and Sami S. David

Not Broken: An Approachable Guide to Miscarriage and Recurrent Pregnancy Loss by Lora Shahine

PCOS SOS: A Gynecologist's Lifeline to Naturally Restore Your Rhythms, Hormones, and Happiness by Felice Gersh and Alexis Perella

The PCOS Workbook: Your Guide to Complete Physical and Emotional Health by Angela Grassi and Stephanie Mattei

Period Power: Harness Your Hormones and Get Your Cycle Working for You by Maisie Hill

Period Repair Manual: Natural Treatment for Better Hormones and Better Periods by Lara Briden

Taking Charge of Your Fertility by Toni Weschler

This Is Your Brain on Birth Control: The Surprising Science of Women, Hormones, and the Law of Unintended Consequences by Sarah Hill

WomanCode: Perfect Your Cycle, Amplify Your Fertility, Supercharge Your Sex Drive, and Become a Power Source by Alisa Vitti

Websites

LoraShahine.com: A fellow fertility specialist and all-around amazing woman, Lora Shahine has not only written a wonderful book and an illustrated counterpart to help couples dealing with miscarriage, but she also discusses books related to fertility on her website.

Bedsider.org

FamilyEquality.org: A website for LGBTQ patients

FertilityForColoredGirls.org

Flo.health

HealthyWomen.org

HelloClue.com

MeetRosy.com

PlannedParenthood.org

ReproductiveFacts.org

Resolve.org: An informative website for infertility advocacy

SimpleHealth.com

TheBrokenBrownEgg.org

Endometriosis

EndoFound.org

EndometriosisAssn.org

PCOS

PCOSAA.org

PCOSChallenge.org

Podcasts

As a Woman: There are many podcasts out there focused on women's health and fertility, but this one, hosted by my colleague Dr. Natalie Crawford, most definitely stands out.

Fertility Friday Radio: Another very good podcast focused on helping women achieve their goals through FAM.

Social Media

Follow me on Instagram at @RKudesia. You will find so many of my amazing colleagues who are similarly offering great content and information to help you better understand your fertility!

References

"Age And Fertility." 2020. Reproductivefacts.Org. ReproductiveFacts.org /news-and-publications/patient-fact-sheets-and-booklets/documents /fact-sheets-and-info-booklets/age-and-fertility.

Boutot, Maegan. 2020. "Natural Birth Control And Fertility Awareness Methods." Helloclue.Com. HelloClue.com/articles/sex /natural-birth-control-fertility-awareness-methods.

"Charting Your Fertility Cycle." 2020. WebMD. WebMD.com/infertility-and -reproduction/fertility-tests-for-women#3-7.

Cooney, Laura G., Iris Lee, Mary D. Sammel, and Anuja Dokras. 2017. "High Prevalence Of Moderate And Severe Depressive And Anxiety Symptoms In Polycystic Ovary Syndrome: A Systematic Review And Meta-Analysis." Human Reproduction 32 (5): 1075–1091. DOI:10.1093/humrep/dex044.

"Creighton Model Fertilitycare™ System." 2020. Creightonmodel.Com. CreightonModel.com/index.html.

"Current Evaluation Of Amenorrhea." 2008. *Fertility And Sterility* 90 (5): S219–S225. DOI:10.1016/j.fertnstert.2008.08.038.

"Definitions Of Infertility And Recurrent Pregnancy Loss: A Committee Opinion." 2020. Fertility And Sterility 113 (3): 533–535. DOI:10.1016/j.fertnstert.2019.11.025.

"Diagnostic Evaluation Of The Infertile Male: A Committee Opinion." 2012. Fertility And Sterility 98 (2): 294–301. DOI:10.1016/j.fertnstert.2012.05.033.

"Diagnostic Evaluation Of The Infertile Female: A Committee Opinion." 2015. Fertility And Sterility 103 (6): e44–e50. DOI:10.1016/j.fertnstert.2015.03.019.

Doyle, Joseph O., Kevin S. Richter, Joshua Lim, Robert J. Stillman, James R. Graham, and Michael J. Tucker. 2016. "Successful Elective And Medically Indicated Oocyte Vitrification And Warming For Autologous In Vitro Fertilization, With Predicted Birth Probabilities For Fertility Preservation According To Number Of Cryopreserved Oocytes And Age At Retrieval." Fertility And Sterility 105 (2): 459–466.e2. DOI:10.1016/j.fertnstert.2015.10.026.

"Endometriosis And Infertility: A Committee Opinion." 2012. Fertility And Sterility 98 (3): 591–598. DOI:10.1016/j.fertnstert.2012.05.031.

"Evaluation And Treatment Of Recurrent Pregnancy Loss: A Committee Opinion."
2012. Fertility And Sterility 98 (5): 1103–1111. DOI:10.1016/j.fertnstert.2012.06.048.

Fauser, Bart C.J.M., Basil C. Tarlatzis, Robert W. Rebar, Richard S. Legro, Adam H.
Balen, Roger Lobo, and Enrico Carmina et al. 2012. "Consensus On Women'S
Health Aspects Of Polycystic Ovary Syndrome (PCOS): The Amsterdam ESHRE
/ASRM-Sponsored 3Rd PCOS Consensus Workshop Group." Fertility And
Sterility 97 (1): 28–38.e25. DOI:10.1016/j.fertnstert.2011.09.024.

"Fertility Awareness Methods | Natural Birth Control." 2020. Plannedparenthood.Org.
PlannedParenthood.org/learn/birth-control/fertility-awareness.

"Getting Pregnant After 35." 2020. WebMD. WebMD.com/baby/pregnant-after-35#1.

Hatcher, Robert A. 2015. Contraceptive Technology. 21st ed. Managing
Contraception LLC.

Husby, Gunhild Kalleberg, Ragnhild Skipnes Haugen, and Mette Haase Moen. 2003.
"Diagnostic Delay In Women With Pain And Endometriosis." Acta Obstetricia Et
Gynecologica Scandinavica 82 (7): 649–653. DOI:10.1034/j.1600-0412.2003.00168.x.

Marino, Jennifer, Tamara Varcoe, Scott Davis, Lisa Moran, Alice Rumbold, Hannah
Brown, Melissa Whitrow, Michael Davies, Vivienne Moore, and Renae Fernandez.
2016. "Fixed Or Rotating Night Shift Work Undertaken By Women: Implications
For Fertility And Miscarriage." Seminars In Reproductive Medicine 34 (02):
074–082. DOI:10.1055/s-0036-1571354.

"Mature Oocyte Cryopreservation: A Guideline." 2013. Fertility And Sterility 99 (1):
37–43. DOI:10.1016/j.fertnstert.2012.09.028.

"Menstruation In Girls And Adolescents: Using The Menstrual Cycle As A Vital
Sign." 2016. Pediatrics 137 (3): e20154480. DOI:10.1542/peds.2015-4480.

"Natural Family Planning And Fertility Awareness." 2020. HHS.Gov. HHS.gov/opa
/pregnancy-prevention/birth-control-methods/natural-family
-planning-and-fertility-awareness/index.html.

Nguyen, Ahn. 2020. SASGOG Pearls Of Exxcellence | The Society For Academic
Specialists In General Obstetrics & Gynecology. Exxcellence.org
/list-of-pearls/post-pill-amenorrhea.

"Obesity And Reproduction: A Committee Opinion." 2015. Fertility And Sterility
104 (5): 1116–1126. DOI:10.1016/j.fertnstert.2015.08.018.

Penzias, Alan, Kristin Bendikson, Samantha Butts, Christos Coutifaris, Tommaso Falcone, Gregory Fossum, and Susan Gitlin et al. 2018. "Diagnostic Evaluation Of Sexual Dysfunction In The Male Partner In The Setting Of Infertility: A Committee Opinion." Fertility And Sterility 110 (5): 833–837. DOI:10.1016/j.fertnstert.2018.07.010.

Petraglia, Felice. 2010. "SOGC Guidelines On Endometriosis: Diagnosis And Management." Journal Of Endometriosis 2 (3): 106–106. DOI:10.1177/228402651000200302.

Pfeifer, Samantha, Samantha Butts, Gregory Fossum, Clarisa Gracia, Andrew La Barbera, Jennifer Mersereau, and Randall Odem et al. 2017. "Optimizing Natural Fertility: A Committee Opinion." Fertility And Sterility 107 (1): 52–58. DOI:10.1016/j.fertnstert.2016.09.029.

Pfister, A., N. Crawford, and A. Steiner. 2019. "The Association Between Ovarian Reserve And Luteal Phase Deficiency." Fertility And Sterility 111 (4): e44. DOI:10.1016/j.fertnstert.2019.02.104.

Piltonen, Terhi T. 2019. "Luteal Phase Deficiency: Are We Chasing A Ghost?" Fertility And Sterility 112 (2): 243–244. DOI:10.1016/j.fertnstert.2019.06.024.

"Polycystic Ovary Syndrome." 2018. Obstetrics & Gynecology 131 (6): e157–e171. DOI:10.1097/aog.0000000000002656.

"Practice Bulletin No. 110: Noncontraceptive Uses Of Hormonal Contraceptives." 2010. Obstetrics & Gynecology 115 (1): 206–218. DOI:10.1097/aog.0b013e3181cb50b5.

"Practice Bulletin No. 128." 2012. Obstetrics & Gynecology 120 (1): 197–206. DOI:10.1097/aog.0b013e318262e320.

"Practice Bulletin No. 136." 2013. Obstetrics & Gynecology 122 (1): 176–185. DOI:10.1097/01.aog.0000431815.52679.bb.

"Practice Bulletin No. 186." 2017. Obstetrics & Gynecology 130 (5): e251–e269. DOI:10.1097/aog.0000000000002400.

"Prepregnancy Counseling." 2019. Fertility And Sterility 111 (1): 32–42. DOI:10.1016/j.fertnstert.2018.12.003.

Speroff, Leon, and Mark Fritz. 2011. Clinical Gynecologic Endocrinology And Infertility. Lippincott, Williams & Wilkins.

Taylor, A. 2003. "Extent Of The Problem." *BMJ* 327 (7412): 434–436. DOI:10.1136
/bmj.327.7412.434.

Teede, Helena J, Marie L Misso, Michael F Costello, Anuja Dokras, Joop Laven, Lisa
Moran, Terhi Piltonen, and Robert J Norman. 2018. "Erratum. Recommendations
From The International Evidence-Based Guideline For The Assessment And
Management Of Polycystic Ovary Syndrome." Human Reproduction 34 (2):
388–388. DOI:10.1093/humrep/dey363.

"Testing And Interpreting Measures Of Ovarian Reserve: A Committee Opinion."
2015. Fertility And Sterility 103 (3): e9–e17. DOI:10.1016/j.fertnstert.2014.12.093.

"The Clinical Relevance Of Luteal Phase Deficiency: A Committee Opinion." 2012.
Fertility And Sterility 98 (5): 1112–1117. DOI:10.1016/j.fertnstert.2012.06.050.

Van Heertum, Kristin, and Brooke Rossi. 2017. "Alcohol And Fertility: How Much Is
Too Much?" Fertility Research And Practice 3 (1). DOI:10.1186/s40738-017-0037-x.

Weschler, Toni. 2015. Taking Charge Of Your Fertility.

Wischmann, T., K. Schilling, B. Toth, S. Rösner, T. Strowitzki, K. Wohlfarth, and H.
Kentenich. 2014. "Sexuality, Self-Esteem And Partnership Quality In Infertile
Women And Men." Geburtshilfe Und Frauenheilkunde 74 (08): 759–763.
DOI:10.1055/s-0034-1368461.

Index

A

Age, 23–24
Anovulatory bleeding, 9
Anti-Müllerian hormone
      (AMH), 5, 17, 23
Apps, fertility, 120

B

Basal body temperature
      (BBT) charting,
      37, 64–70, 115
Beta-human chorionic
      gonadotropin
      (β-hCG), 7, 10
Billings, John, 39
Billings Ovulation Method
      (BOM), 39, 61
Birth control, 28–30
Breastfeeding, and
      charting, 116

C

Calendar methods, 46–50
Cervical mucus monitoring,
      54–55, 57–60
Cervical positioning, 56
Charting
   apps and websites, 120
   basal body temperature
      (BBT), 37, 64–70
   blank charts, 128–139
   calendar methods,
      46–50
   cervical mucus, 54–60

endometriosis
      sample, 101–103
   frequently asked
      questions, 115–116
   miscarriage sample, 109–111
   ovarian reserve
      diminishment
      sample, 105–107
   PCOS sample, 97–99
   reading conflicting
      signs, 112–113
   samples, 74–95
   starting a new
      chart, 113–114
Contraception, 28–30
Corpus luteum, 6, 18
Creighton Model, 39, 61
CycleBeads bracelet, 49
Cysts, 18, 21

D

Depo-Provera shot, 28, 30
Dysmenorrhea, 19, 20

E

Eggs, 3
Endometriosis, 19–22,
      70, 101–103
Endometrium, 9–10
Estrogen, 6, 10. *See also*
      Hormonal birth control

F

Fallopian tubes, 19–21
Feldman, Barbara, 39

Fertility awareness methods
      (FAM). *See also* Charting
   about, 36–37, 41
   case studies, 31–32, 41–42
   cons, 40–41
   history of, 39
   hormone testing, 121–123
   pros, 40
   transitioning from
      hormonal birth
      control to, 37–38
Fertility monitors, 122
Fertility preservation, 24
Fertility specialists, 124–125
Follicles, 3
Follicle-stimulating hormone
      (FSH), 6, 28, 122
Follicular phase, 5–6

G

Geriatric pregnancy, 23
Gonadotropin-releasing
      hormone (GnRH), 6

H

Hillebrand, Wilhelm, 39
Hormonal birth control,
      28–30, 37–38, 116
Hormones. *See specific*
Hormone testing, 121–123
Hyperandrogenism, 16
Hyperthyroidism, 25
Hypothalamus, 4–5
Hypothyroidism, 25

I

Infertility diagnosis, 14
Intrauterine devices
(IUDs), 28, 30

K

Knaus, Hermann, 39

L

Long-acting reversible
contraceptives
(LARCs), 30
Luteal phase, 6–8
Luteal phase defect (LPD), 8
Luteinizing hormone (LH),
6, 36, 61, 112, 121–122

M

Male infertility, 14–15
Marquette Method, 39, 61, 122
Menstrual cycle
about, 3
duration, 4
as the "fifth vital sign," 2
ovarian cycle, 4–8
uterine cycle, 9–10
Menstruation, 9
Miscarriage, 26–27, 109–111
Mittelschmerz, 6

N

NaPro Technology, 39

O

Ogino, Kyusaku, 39
Oral contraceptive pills
(OCPs), 18–19, 21, 28–29

Ovarian cycle, 4–7
Ovarian reserve, 3, 5,
70, 105–107
Ovarian torsion, 18
Ovulation, 6, 16, 36–37, 115
Ovulation predictor kits
(OPKs), 121–122

P

Periods, 9
Pituitary gland, 5
Polycystic ovary syndrome
(PCOS), 9, 16–19,
60, 69, 97–99
Pregnancy loss, 26–27
Premenstrual dysphoric
disorder (PMDD), 7
Premenstrual syndrome
(PMS), 7
Progesterone, 6–10, 65.
See also Hormonal
birth control
Prolactin, 5
Proliferative phase, 10

R

Reproductive system, 2
Retrograde menstruation, 19
Rock, John, 39
Rotterdam criteria, 16–17

S

Saliva ferning, 123
Secretory phase, 10
Semen analysis, 15
Sexual dysfunction, 15

Smulders, Johannes, 39
Standard Days Method
(SDM), 39, 48–50

T

Temperature tracking. *See*
Basal body temperature
(BBT) charting
Testosterone, 15, 16
Thermometers, 122
Thyroid issues, 25, 70
Thyroid-stimulating
hormone (TSH), 25
Thyrotropin-releasing
hormone (TRH), 25

U

Uterine cycle, 9–10

V

Vaginal discharge, 60.
See also Cervical
mucus monitoring
Velde, Theodoor Hendrik
Van de, 39

W

Wearable devices, 122
Websites, fertility, 120
Weschler, Toni, 39
World Organisation of
Ovulation Method
Billings (WOOMB), 61

Acknowledgments

Though the process of writing a book takes time, it is often the case—and definitely true for me—that the years of gaining the knowledge presented in said book are by far the bigger undertaking. Thank you so much to Katie Parr, Mo Mozuch, and the Callisto team for entrusting me with this book. Writing it has only fueled my appreciation for how truly intricate the process of reproduction is.

Having reached the point of authoring this first book, I have so many individuals I want to thank for their support along the way. From an educational standpoint, I have been blessed to have more standout educators in my life than I can count. In high school, Julie Winter, Anne Sandoval, and Marc Fazio were three teachers who believed in me even while I was still seeking my own confidence and path. In college, Anne Fausto-Sterling set me on the path to a career in reproductive medicine, who challenged me to always write better and more succinctly, and to remember the impact of science, particularly of assisted reproductive technologies, on society. My RJT crew—Angela Feraco, Tara Ramchandani, Susannah Raub, and Jen Rosenbaum—you are friends for life, and inspirations to keep living my dreams.

My medical school years were full of people who modeled the kind of physician I aspired to be—compassionate, thoughtful, evidence-based—and those who reminded me that the privilege of a premier education comes with assuming the mantle of leadership, and pushing medicine forward. Annie Lyerly enriched my understanding of the nuances of clinical women's healthcare, risk perception in pregnancy, and the realities of life as an OB/GYN and a physician mother. Conversations with Kathy Rudy helped me continue to link reproductive medicine with feminism and women's studies. Jeff Wilkinson also taught me much about real-world OB/GYN, and his guidance led me to unforgettable clinical experiences in settings as disparate as the Navajo Nation and Niger. Supriya Rao and Mike Rhodes, thank you for all the journeys we shared during these years and beyond.

In seven years of residency and fellowship training, when a newly minted doctor is forged into a physician (often through the fire of hazing and sleep deprivation), I was lucky to have some amazing fellow physicians in my life. I may not have made it through the journey to become an obstetrician-gynecologist without my coresidents and close friends, Bani Ratan, Jamie Kramer, and Raeka Talati, to whom I could easily pen an ode of gratitude. My mentors, Mike Worley, Steve Chasen, and Divya Gupta all helped me see the difficulty of balancing research with clinical practice, and yet how rewarding the quest can be, and especially how important it is to follow the data and not simply be dragged in and out with the tide of the status quo.

From my fellowship years, I am grateful beyond words to Harry Lieman, Staci Pollack, and Erkan Buyuk, who molded me into the fertility specialist I am today. I am grateful for your ongoing mentorship and friendship. Beth McAvey, my ASRM roomie, thank you for being a friend, a supporter, and a role model, and for helping me follow you from residency to fellowship to our years together at RMA. Joe Davis and Peter Klatsky, your friendships couldn't have come at a better time—I learned so much from your perspectives and all the hours discussing medicine and life.

After completing my training, I have had the fortune of two amazing jobs. To my team at the Reproductive Medicine Associates of New York: what an unforgettable three years. Simply put, I learned so much and had a great time doing so (Team BK forever!). I miss everything but the frenetic pace and the endless emails! Alan Copperman, thank you for taking me under your wing, providing me so many opportunities for growth, and teaching me what inspirational leadership looks like. Your mentorship and personal support mean the world.

And to my team at CCRM Fertility Houston, I am so glad that I landed here and get to spend the rest of my career working with y'all, locally and across our entire network. Our team is phenomenal. To work with pioneers in the field like Bill Schoolcraft, Mandy Katz-Jaffe, and my colleagues across our international network is a dream come true. In Colorado, Jon, Scott, and Alison: thank you for being so supportive of my forward growth. Constance, Jen, and Jordan—you are a trio always bestowing me with amazing PR gifts and I appreciate the trust you place in me to spread the CCRM message far and wide. In Houston, I could easily list our entire staff in gratitude (y'all are just that good!), but Susan, I don't think I would make it a week without you—thank you for all you do. Shout-out to my Sugar Land team: Nikki, Thessa, Ashly—please, don't ever leave me! A deep and heartfelt thank-you to my partners, Tim Hickman, Jamie Nodler, and especially Katherine McKnight, for bringing me on to the team, cheerleading my growth, and helping me navigate this new world of parenthood as a physician.

As I gain years of experience in medicine, I feel increasingly humble about how much my patients teach me. Through unique twists in their family-building story, the emotional connection we build along the way, the scientifically challenging cases, all of it—thank you for entrusting me to guide one of the most personal roller coasters that we ever ride as human beings. It is such an honor to be on this journey alongside each and every one of you.

I also realize more and more how much of a toll a calling to medicine takes on those we love in our personal lives. I am endlessly grateful to my family. To my parents, Vijay and Alka Kudesia, who wisely tried to warn me about the sacrifice inherent to this work but nonetheless tirelessly supported me and celebrated every accolade and achievement along the way. To my brother, Ravi, my very first best friend and life coach—thank you for always being there for me. And to my husband, Ashish, who stuck with me even when you realized that "I don't work that much" was completely delusional—thank you for being on this journey with me, with all its ups and downs, and for growing a family and becoming a better person with me. Through you, I am also so lucky to have experienced the love of your parents, whose support I have both in person and in spirit. And to the two little rascals who fill me with peace, love, and sometimes extreme exhaustion, my dearest Amara and Bowser. The cuddles and looks of love you give embody why humans crave family, and what urges women to consider undergoing all the techniques and approaches discussed in this book. In life, you are my why, and I love you.

About the Author

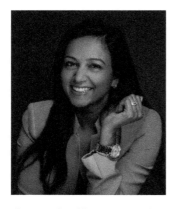

Rashmi Kudesia, MD, MSc, is a board-certified reproductive endocrinologist and infertility specialist at CCRM Fertility Houston in Houston, Texas, where she serves as the director of patient education and Sugar Land site director. She is also the assistant clinical professor of OB/GYN at Houston Methodist Hospital, the medical director for Simple Health, and a member of the board of directors of Planned Parenthood Gulf Coast.

Dr. Kudesia was born in Chicago and grew up in suburban Detroit before moving to Rhode Island, where she received her Sc.B. in biology and medicine magna cum laude from Brown University, followed by her MD with honors from the Duke University School of Medicine. She then pursued OB/GYN residency at the New York-Presbyterian/Weill Cornell Medical Center, followed by an REI fellowship at the Albert Einstein College of Medicine, Montefiore, while earning her MSc in clinical research methods. She subsequently served as a clinical assistant professor at the Icahn School of Medicine at Mount Sinai before relocating to Houston, where she currently resides with her husband, daughter, and very spoiled labradoodle, Bowser.

Dr. Kudesia has held many national leadership roles in organized medicine, allowing her to advance and advocate for women's health through positions within the American Society of Reproductive Medicine, the American Medical Association, and more. She has received multiple grants and awards for her scientific research, which she has published and presented widely. Both her research and advocacy focus on access to fertility knowledge, counseling and care, polycystic ovary syndrome, and LGBTQ fertility. She promotes reproductive health and empowerment through various advisory board appointments and community outreach as well as on social media platforms, including Facebook and Instagram (@RKudesia), and Twitter (@RashmiKudesia).

CPSIA information can be obtained
at www.ICGtesting.com
Printed in the USA
LVHW070035011020
667550LV00029B/685

9 781647 393564